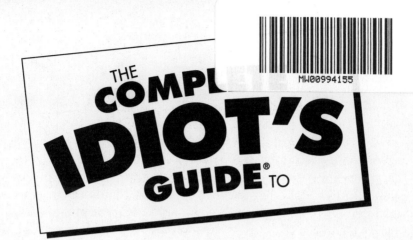

THE COMPLETE IDIOT'S GUIDE® TO

Detoxing Your Body

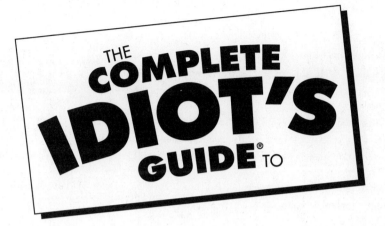

THE COMPLETE **IDIOT'S** GUIDE® TO

Detoxing Your Body

by Delia Quigley

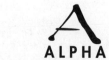

ALPHA

A member of Penguin Group (USA) Inc.

ALPHA BOOKS

Published by the Penguin Group

Penguin Group (USA) Inc., 375 Hudson Street, New York, New York 10014, USA

Penguin Group (Canada), 90 Eglinton Avenue East, Suite 700, Toronto, Ontario M4P 2Y3, Canada (a division of Pearson Penguin Canada Inc.)

Penguin Books Ltd, 80 Strand, London WC2R 0RL, England

Penguin Ireland, 25 St. Stephen's Green, Dublin 2, Ireland (a division of Penguin Books Ltd.)

Penguin Group (Australia), 250 Camberwell Road, Camberwell, Victoria 3124, Australia (a division of Pearson Australia Group Pty. Ltd.)

Penguin Books India Pvt. Ltd., 11 Community Centre, Panchsheel Park, New Delhi—110 017, India

Penguin Group (NZ), 67 Apollo Drive, Rosedale, North Shore, Auckland 1311, New Zealand (a division of Pearson New Zealand Ltd.)

Penguin Books (South Africa) (Pty.) Ltd, 24 Sturdee Avenue, Rosebank, Johannesburg 2196, South Africa

Penguin Books Ltd., Registered Offices: 80 Strand, London WC2R 0RL, England

Copyright © 2008 by Delia Quigley

International Standard Book Number: 978-1-59257-720-0
Library of Congress Catalog Card Number: Available upon request

12 11 10   8 7 6 5 4

Interpretation of the printing code: The rightmost number of the first series of numbers is the year of the book's printing; the rightmost number of the second series of numbers is the number of the book's printing. For example, a printing code of 08-1 shows that the first printing occurred in 2008.

Printed in the United States of America

Most Alpha books are available at special quantity discounts for bulk purchases for sales promotions, premiums, fund-raising, or educational use. Special books, or book excerpts, can also be created to fit specific needs.

For details, write: Special Markets, Alpha Books, 375 Hudson Street, New York, NY 10014.

Publisher: *Marie Butler-Knight*
Editorial Director/Acquiring Editor: *Mike Sanders*
Managing Editor: *Billy Fields*
Development Editor: *Lynn Northrup*
Production Editor: *Kayla Dugger*
Copy Editor: *Amy Borelli*

Cartoonist: *Steve Barr*
Cover Designer: *Bill Thomas*
Book Designer: *Trina Wurst*
Indexer: *Brad Herriman*
Layout: *Brian Massey*
Proofreader: *Aaron Black*

In memory of Dr. Wally Burnstein. He spoke for those who could not speak; he spoke for those who would not speak.

Contents at a Glance

Contents

Foreword

Often, when new clients come to me with stories of their attempts at a detoxification program, I cringe inwardly, knowing that I most likely will be asked to help them undo some negative effects that resulted from that effort. Many have learned, the hard way, that detoxifying before the body has been properly prepared can lead to a very unsatisfactory outcome.

But help is at hand. Delia Quigley explains why and how one should build up nutritionally before attempting to detoxify. She directs us to the healthy foods necessary for the build-up while pointing out the toxic foods and chemicals that should be avoided. This is key for the success of a detoxification program. Encouraging the body to release its store of toxins while continuing to add more toxins can sabotage any cleansing effort. By the same token, detoxifying a body with a blocked colon or cleansing faster than the body's ability to manage can impair detoxification efforts and leave one feeling worse than before. These potential pitfalls can be avoided by following the detoxification program outlined by Delia.

She shows you how to intelligently prepare the body for a detox by identifying the "correct" foods while pinpointing damaging foods and toxins. Next, Delia leads you to the crux of detoxing: a short, controlled fast followed by the gradual resumption of eating foods that will serve to maintain new-found health.

Eyes will brighten, brains will clear, skin will glow, weight will balance, and moods will soar after Delia Quigley's detoxifying program. She offers us a life-altering experience that empowers us with the knowledge to manage health and extend longevity. Thank you, Delia.

I wish you luck and good health.

Dian Freeman
Certified in Clinical Nutrition and Holistic Health
www.dianshealthandherbs.com

Introduction

If we were to make a movie of the day in the life of an average American, the opening shot might show you reluctant to get up out of bed. The day looms ahead and you are feeling heavy and bloated, your skin has a gray tinge, and your back is killing you again. You manage to swing your legs over the side of the bed, but when you stand up pain suddenly shoots across the soles of your feet and up your legs. You quickly sit back down, place your head into your hands, and wonder how it all came to this.

You've been to your doctor numerous times, and he or she has you taking medication for high blood pressure and elevated levels of cholesterol, antidepressants, and pain killers. All these pills, all that money out of pocket, and still you feel like you've been run over by a truck. There has got to be another way, you think, yet you have no idea what to do.

"If I could just clean everything out and start fresh," you say to yourself, "like when I was a kid with all that energy and spontaneity. I feel old and sick and my life is passing me by."

The camera pans back as you stand once again and we see you as you are: distended belly, slumped shoulders, bags under your eyes, and 40 pounds overweight. You catch sight of yourself in the mirror and realize for the first time, "I need to clean my body from the inside out."

You are now ready to detoxify your body.

It has only been in the past 50 years that human beings have trashed the earth so badly that detoxification of our vital body systems is necessary for healthy survival. Our food supply has undergone rigorous transformations from the organic, farm-fresh ingredients of four generations ago to processed foods lacking nutrients and vitality. This refined, chemical-laden diet has resulted in a multitude of diseases known only to our present-day Western civilization.

According to physician and activist Dr. Wally Burnstein, D.O., "If everybody has cancer, if children are developing cancer at the age of 5 and 10 years old, then we're destroying our future generations, our gonadal tissue, our DNA, so all future generations will have birth defects, everybody's born with birth defects, so what's the sense, nothing else is more important, nothing takes precedence over detoxifying our bodies, preserving our food supply and protecting our Mother Earth."

The human species is presently the most frail, fragile species the earth has ever seen. The horizontally ill are in bed; you know they're sick because they are lying in bed unable to get up. The vertically ill are up walking around. Americans are walking around with digestive problems, autoimmune diseases, cancer, diabetes, and other chronic illnesses. Americans are the vertically ill, but it doesn't have to be this way. Eating an organic whole-foods diet with consistent periods of detoxification will go a long way toward healing you and the planet. This is what these times are calling for. Reading this book is the first step toward protecting your health and the health of your family.

How to Use This Book

The Complete Idiot's Guide to Detoxing Your Body is divided into five parts:

Part 1, "You Need to Detox!," tells you why detoxing is the future of all dietary programs. In order to continue to stay healthy in our chemical-driven culture, everyone will need to detoxify. Fill out the questionnaires in Chapter 1 and you will learn how toxic you are and where in your environment those toxins are coming from. Then find out how detoxing cleanses your filtering organs, glands, and bloodstream, which results in more energy, vitality, clarity of mind, and a positive outlook on life.

Part 2, "Preparing to Detoxify," shows you all the essentials you will need, from supplements to cleansing products, food, teas, and encouragement for making your detox program a complete success. You will also learn about the side effects that can occur when eliminating toxins and chemicals from your body.

Part 3, "Ladies and Gentlemen, Start Your Organs," is the ultimate detox program laid out over a five-week period—two weeks to prepare, one week to fast, and two weeks to complete the detoxification. Perfect for everyone who needs to change their diet, improve their health, and achieve overall feelings of lightness and well-being.

Part 4, "Alternative Detox Choices," details short, effective detoxification programs that target specific health problems you may be experiencing. A spring fling, gastrointestinal problems, and a gallbladder flush are all addressed in these inspiring chapters. Then there is the weekend getaway that will transform you in just a matter of days.

Part 5, "Mind, Body, and Spirit," shows how there is more to detoxifying than just flushing your organs. When you pamper yourself with relaxing baths and facials, open your pores and let the toxins pour out, and calm your mind with yoga and meditation, you are seeing to the whole being and not just a small part. This is the part that will help ease your way through the dietary changes and speed the process, making your detoxification more effective.

Detoxifying Knowledge in a Box

You'll also find four different types of sidebars throughout the chapters that supplement the text:

Healthy Tidbits

These boxes provide you with interesting tips, information, comments, and stories about detoxifying that will make your detox program go more smoothly.

Pure Insights

These quotes from medical, nutritional, environmental, and spiritual experts put an interesting spin on the subject of detoxification.

Detox Alert

Here you'll find warning signs, tips for when to use caution, and things to look out for.

def•i•ni•tion

Check out these boxes for definitions of words and terms that you may not be familiar with.

Acknowledgments

My thanks to Lorraine Fasano for all her generous help and support. To Lucinda Amodio for her menu contributions, Maria Prinz for her essential oil information, and Susan Jalbert and Alice Smith for their editing assistance.

To the editing staff at Alpha Books, my thanks for putting the manuscript into shape; and to Lynn Northrup and Mike Sanders for your patient guidance during the writing process.

Special Thanks to the Technical Reviewers

The Complete Idiot's Guide to Detoxing Your Body was reviewed by Dr. Dana Cohen, M.D., and Dr. Rashmi Gulati, M.D. Their expert review of the manuscript ensures that the information provided in this book is accurate and effective for you to practice. You can view their website at www.patientsmedical.com.

Dr. Cohen is board certified by the American Board of Internal Medicine. She received her medical degree from St. George's University School of Medicine in Grenada, West Indies, and completed her residency at Albany Medical Center in Albany, New York.

Dr. Cohen has recently joined Patients Medical in New York City, a comprehensive medical center specializing in integrating holistic and alternative therapies with western medicine. Dr. Cohen focuses on nutrition and preventative medicine while incorporating the best of allopathic and integrative medicine modalities. She also has expertise in male and female hormone replacement therapy.

Dr. Gulati, graduated among the top of her class from Rohtak Medical College with a Master's degree in pathology. She then studied and graduated with a Master's in internal medicine, and has trained as a holistic physician with the American College for Advancement in Medicine. Dr. Gulati took over as medical director of Patients Medical Integrative and Internal Medicine in New York City in 2004. Dr. Gulati has specialized in both internal and integrative medicine and with her allopathic clinical experience enhanced by her naturopathic expertise is able to truly integrate both disciplines.

Trademarks

All terms mentioned in this book that are known to be or are suspected of being trademarks or service marks have been appropriately capitalized. Alpha Books and Penguin Group (USA) Inc. cannot attest to the accuracy of this information. Use of a term in this book should not be regarded as affecting the validity of any trademark or service mark.

Part 1

You Need to Detox!

Detoxing your body is the latest diet phenomenon to hit America. It is being touted as the most important and beneficial health treatment you can do for yourself. Not just a diet for weight loss, "detoxing" cleanses your filtering organs, glands, and bloodstream, which results in more energy, vitality, clarity of mind, and a positive outlook on life. It is also a wonderful rejuvenator for tired and aging skin.

In this part, you will find out just how toxic you are, what is causing the problem, and what you will need to start feeling better. Even with a healthy diet and lifestyle, you'll be surprised with just how hard it is to stay clean in today's world.

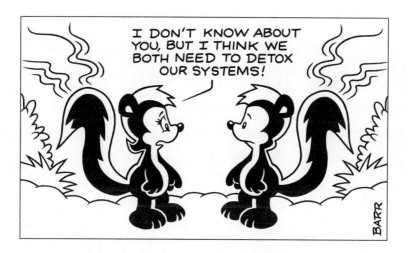

I Need to *What?*

In This Chapter

- ◆ What is detoxing?
- ◆ Why you should detox
- ◆ How "toxic" are you?
- ◆ Understanding food intolerance, allergies, and sensitivities
- ◆ The benefits of detoxing

The catch phrase for the twenty-first century should be, "You need to detox!" It should be spoken with just the right amount of vocal concern and just a bit of needling. And no wonder. Scientists have been finding toxic levels of pollutants in our food, air, and the water we drink. They have also found them in our blood, fat, organs, urine, and even breast milk. You have no idea how many poisons you are absorbing into your system on a daily basis. The good news is you can rid your body of these toxins with a good detox program.

In this chapter, you will learn what it means to detox, find out why detoxing is beneficial for your health, and take a look at just how toxic you really are.

The Detox Lowdown

Detoxification is what happens when you improve the quality of the food you eat, change your lifestyle for the better, and/or give up some bad habits. The reason you do this is to feel better in your physical body, and ultimately to feel better about yourself. Detoxing is something everyone can and should do at least once a year—especially if you are experiencing any of these often-debilitating symptoms:

- Low-grade or migraine headaches
- Digestive problems
- Gas and bloating
- Irritable bowel syndrome
- Muscular aches and pains
- Gastrointestinal problems
- Depression
- Immune weakness
- Persistent fatigue
- Inability to lose weight

def•i•ni•tion

Detoxification is the metabolic process by which toxins are changed into less toxic or more readily excretable substances.

If you suffer from any of these symptoms, I suggest you take the Lifestyle questionnaire later in this chapter to find out how toxic you really are.

Why Should You Detox?

Whether you are in good health, feeling run down, or exhibiting symptoms of illness, it's always a good idea to take time to detoxify your internal system. For starters, you will end up looking and feeling fabulous. If that's not motivation enough, consider the scientific research showing how important it is to detoxify the many chemicals and toxins we encounter each day. Your body is detoxing all the time, but if you cannot do this naturally (and some people cannot), it can lead to debilitating illnesses. Drugs, hormones, and heavy metals can build up in your system when it's not detoxifying properly. Chronic fatigue syndrome, fibromyalgia, and multiple chemical sensitivities are related to this. There is also a link between chronic neurological diseases (Parkinson's) and certain types of cancer that stem from a person's inability to naturally detoxify.

Besides toxins and chemicals, what is there left to detox? According to the supplement company Nature's Sunshine, Inc., in one year the average American will consume:

- 150 slices of pizza
- 566 cans of soda
- 150 pounds of sugar
- 45 large bags of potato chips
- 120 orders of French fries
- 190 large candy bars
- 120 pastries or desserts

This is a tremendous amount of refined sugar, hydrogenated fats, food additives, and nutrient-lacking foods. This way of eating can be the cause of many of the symptoms you have been experiencing.

Your digestive and intestinal system can detoxify a portion of your daily food intake, but after years or even decades of eating a high-fat, refined-flour diet, your body cannot keep up with the onslaught. Your precision body systems were not designed to function on refined flour and sugar for an entire lifetime. They will need *your* attention along the way. Think "detox" and then take action!

Healthy Tidbits

You probably take better care of your car then you do your body. Every 3,000 to 6,000 miles, you take your car to the shop to get its oil and filter changed, tires checked and rotated, fluids topped, inside vacuumed, and chrome polished. Your body also needs its filtering organs changed, fluids cleaned, and joints oiled to keep it running like a smooth machine. Periodically detoxing can take care of this for you.

Your Amazing Body

Unbeknownst to you, your body is detoxifying all the time. This makes sense given that your body is geared to do one thing and one thing only—and that is to survive.

Despite the many harrowing adventures you put it through—all the junk food, sugar, caffeine, and alcohol you will consume in a lifetime—your body will do its best to survive. Detoxification is one of the most important ways in which your body will attempt to pull this off.

The natural intelligence of your body has its hands full dealing with the unlimited number of bizarre and exotic chemicals you ingest daily. This is all happening while your body makes sure your lungs take in oxygen; your digestive system breaks down and eliminates food; your pancreas has enough insulin to counter the candy bar, soda, and cheese doodles you just consumed; and your insatiable brain is fed enough nutrients.

Your body knows that your cells are in danger of being damaged by the toxins and chemicals we explore in Chapter 2. Damaged cells weaken the immune system, opening the way for disease to enter. Detoxification can help prevent this from happening.

The difference between the medical *allopathic* approach and the *complementary* health approach is the former favors addressing one symptom, giving one diagnosis, and offering one drug to "cure" or "suppress" the symptom. The complementary approach is to see the body as a whole entity and foster natural remedies that are less disruptive to the body's ecology. Dr. Dana Cohen of Patients Medical, a holistic and integrative clinic in New York City, believes "It is my philosophy to do everything in my power to keep patients off of medications, and that using a medication is a last resort. Whereas, more often than not, an allopathic physician uses medication as a first line [of] therapy."

The Process of Survival

No, it's not time to discuss that form of elimination—not yet, anyway. (I introduce that most delicate of subjects, bowel elimination, in Chapter 7, so stay tuned.) For now let us return to that survival instinct I mentioned earlier. Your body deals with dangerous substances floating around the bloodstream by storing them in your fatty tissue. It is your body's job to convert these fat-soluble toxins into water-soluble, nontoxic metabolites and discharge them through your organs of elimination. This prevents a buildup of toxins in your blood, which can lead to internal poisoning of the entire system. Pretty smart, eh?

Problems arise when the body cannot keep up with your toxic lifestyle. Overwhelmed and with no outside help, your body will find other ways to get rid of the poisons. Colds are one way the body eliminates excess mucus and toxins. Now, if you are like most people, you won't go to bed and rest. You will take an over-the-counter cold medication, go to work, and sit at your desk feeling awful. Your co-workers will try to avoid you because they don't want to have to detoxify the germs you are sneezing into the air. The cold medication you took will only suppress the symptoms and drive the cause deeper into your body. You want all that runny, sweaty stuff to come out, not dive back into your overtaxed system.

With periodic detoxing, as outlined in this book, you will learn how to work with your body rather than against it. You will have fewer colds, and your immune system will strengthen. All your systems will be working as they should, clean and efficiently.

Toxins in Your Body

I will use the word *toxins* to describe any poisonous substance that accumulates in the body. These poisons can include the following:

- Bacterial organisms
- Environmental chemicals
- Trans fatty acids
- Parasites
- Herbicides and pesticides
- Viral organisms
- Candida albicans (an overgrowth of yeast organisms in the large intestine; discussed in Chapter 4)
- Heavy metals

def•i•ni•tion

> **Toxins** are any poison substances in your body that cause harm and destroy your health. When your body is weak and overburdened with toxins, the organs of elimination cannot excrete properly, resulting in the accumulation of body waste. In other words, if you don't take out the garbage, your house is going to become a smelly mess.

Can I Work and Detox?

The five-week detox program I outline in this book can be done while you are working. Your major consideration will be to make sure you bring a lunch prepared according to the detox menu. (Chapter 5 will guide you in how to order meals in restaurants.) You'll still find plenty to eat, although you may have to put up with a few snide remarks from your co-workers about what you are eating.

During the fasting week, try to coordinate your fast with a weekend when you can stay close to home and just relax. I have known people who work at their desk all day, so drinking liquids was not difficult to do. However, for the best results, fasting days should be done in a relaxing atmosphere without pressure or food temptations around you. Believe me when I say that while fasting, you can smell a pizza a mile away!

Getting a Checkup

As with any new dietary program, I suggest you consult your doctor and get a thorough checkup before starting the detox program. This way you can compare your cholesterol and high blood pressure levels before and after detoxing. Your doctor will be aware of what you are doing and help monitor any reactions you might experience. When you follow the detox instructions outlined in Part 3, you will be amazed at how your body will rebalance and regulate itself when given the proper nutrition.

Just How Toxic Are You?

Let's say after taking every medical test, you have no answer for those unexplained symptoms. You were told it is all in your head—except those aches and pains aren't going away. The brain fog and fatigue are ruining your life. No one can tell you what is wrong, and the medication only makes things worse. You need to detox!

Detox Alert

The results of these questionnaires should not be used to diagnose or treat a medical condition. Take them with you when consulting your doctor so he or she can better assess your condition.

Blood tests are very useful for diagnostic purposes. Given that your blood is the river that runs through every part of your body, it's going to give a pretty good indication of what's happening on the inside. However, the diagnostician will need some extra information to pinpoint the cause of your difficulties.

In the questionnaires that follow, you will have the chance to identify all those odd aches and pains you've been feeling, take a look at your surrounding environment, and discover just what you've been living with.

Lifestyle Questionnaire

These questions are just for you to answer. No one else ever has to see the results, if you wish. The questions cover a lot of ground and will probably have you thinking about your lifestyle in ways you never have before. They are designed to cover all areas of exposure to processed foods, refined sugar, soda pop, prescription and/or recreational drugs, and environmental chemicals.

Place a checkmark next to those choices that relate to your lifestyle. At the end of the list, add up your checkmarks and evaluate your score.

Do you eat or drink the following at least three or four times per week?

- ❑ Black tea or coffee
- ❑ Sodas or diet sodas
- ❑ Convenience or processed meals or foods
- ❑ White bread, pasta, rice, and pastries
- ❑ Snack foods: chips, pretzels, cookies, cakes
- ❑ Foods containing artificial sweeteners
- ❑ Smoked foods (bacon, fish, cheese, meats)
- ❑ Barbecued food
- ❑ Nonorganic fruit (without washing and peeling first)
- ❑ Nonorganic green vegetables (without removing outer leaves)
- ❑ Nonorganic root vegetables (without scrubbing and peeling)
- ❑ Processed meats (sausages, burgers, hot dogs, etc.)
- ❑ Fried foods
- ❑ Iodized salt
- ❑ More than two glasses of alcohol per day
- ❑ Ice cream and/or frozen yogurt

Do you:

- ❑ Live in a city?
- ❑ Live within a mile of a major road?
- ❑ Live under a busy flight path?
- ❑ Live near a power station or within half a mile of high-voltage overhead power cables?

- ❑ Often walk or run along busy roads?
- ❑ Live near fields that are regularly sprayed with pesticides?
- ❑ Often swim in a pool containing chlorinated water?
- ❑ Use a cell phone?
- ❑ Have central heating or air conditioning?
- ❑ Use synthetic air fresheners?
- ❑ Use pesticides in your house or garden?
- ❑ Use large amounts of bleach, detergent, household cleaners, or disinfectant?
- ❑ Work with a computer?
- ❑ Smoke cigarettes?
- ❑ Use recreational drugs on a regular basis?
- ❑ Use prescription or over-the-counter drugs on a regular basis?
- ❑ Cook or heat your house with gas-powered appliances?
- ❑ Have your clothes dry-cleaned regularly?
- ❑ Have much chipboard, fiberboard, or plywood in your house?
- ❑ Have plumbing in your home more than 20 years old?

Have you:

- ❑ Recently had your house treated for woodworm, termites, or rot, or put in new timber?
- ❑ Recently bought soft furnishings, especially those with "stain resistant" finishes?
- ❑ Recently laid new carpet or vinyl flooring?
- ❑ Recently repainted the interior of your house?

If you checked:

Less than 10: Although your lifestyle is pretty healthy, the five-week detox program will do you good and keep you healthy.

Between 11–20: You are exposed to toxic chemicals at an average level. The detox program can easily reduce your total toxic load.

More than 21: You are consistently exposed to toxic chemicals in your food and environment. You will need to take time to detox slowly, but following the detox program is necessary.

The questions you answered cover a broad spectrum of exposures to chemicals and other toxins. It may have been a real eye-opener to see how many things in your life are considered toxic in some form. It is the price we pay for living with the technology we have created.

Healthy Tidbits _____

Scientists speculate that 100 years from now we will have found a way to preserve nature and sustain a healthy population. Humans of the future will look back on our culture amazed at our willingness to pollute the air, food, and water meant to sustain our lives. By detoxing your body and changing your lifestyle, you can reduce the toxic load we all carry into the future.

Sensitivities Questionnaire

With all that exposure to chemicals, toxins, and a stress-filled life, you may have developed a few sensitivities to certain smells, tastes, and body products. This next set of questions is designed to get you thinking about how you react to many of the products you encounter. Check all that apply.

Do you have a negative reaction to any of the following:

❑ Chemicals, car fumes, odors, perfumes, or fragrances

❑ Caffeine, alcohol, or medications

❑ Monosodium glutamate (MSG)

❑ Foods containing sulfites, such as wine and dried fruit, or salad bar food

❑ Diet sodas containing artificial sweeteners

Do you suffer from any of these symptoms:

❑ Fibromayalgia, chronic fatigue syndrome, cancer, or an autoimmune disease

❑ Acne, eczema, hives, or general itching

❑ Fatigue, lethargy, joint pains, muscle aches, or weakness

❑ Mood swings, anxiety, depression, poor concentration, a "spacey" feeling, or restlessness

❏ Headaches, sinus infections, or allergies

❏ Nausea, bad breath, foul-smelling stools, a bloated feeling, or intolerance to fatty or starchy foods

Most importantly, do you keep getting sick?

If you checked three or more, the five-week detox program in this book is very important for you because you may be displaying signs of toxicity. You need to detoxify your body and decrease your exposure to chemicals and toxins.

Symptoms Questionnaire

There are certain physical symptoms you live with; some disrupt your life, while others you tolerate without question. You've learned to live with them. This next questionnaire is about the symptoms you live with day to day and the ones that show up out of nowhere, last a week or a few days, and then disappear again.

Just before you begin your detox program, fill in the questionnaire, total the numbers, then set it aside. Upon completion of your five-week program repeat the questionnaire and compare the two scores. Notice what symptoms have changed or no longer exist. Notice, too, what symptoms are still present; this will show you that there's still more detoxification you can do to improve your health.

Place a number before each symptom that best describes its severity. Enter 1 for very mild and 10 for very severe. Enter 0 if no symptoms are present.

_____ Flulike symptoms

_____ Dark circles under eyes

_____ Muscle aches and pains

_____ Swollen glands

_____ Shortness of breath

_____ Muscle weakness

_____ Numbness, tingling, burning

_____ Burning, tearing eyes

_____ Hair loss

_____ Vertigo

_____ Metallic body odor

_____ A feeling of "what's the use?"

_____ Cough, lung infection

_____ Sinus trouble

_____ Sore throat

_____ Bladder infections

_____ Fever

_____ Craving breads/carbs

_____ Craving sugar/alcohol

_____ Postnasal drip

_____ Coated tongue

_____ Symptoms are worse in damp weather

_____ Dry, burning, metallic mouth

_____ Ear pain, itching

_____ Burning urination

_____ Athlete's foot/nail fungus

_____ Vaginal or penile itching/burning

_____ Fungus

_____ Sensitive to tobacco smoke

_____ Rashes

_____ Sensitive to smells and odor

_____ Yeasty body odor

_____ Confusion/poor concentration

_____ Lack of balance

_____ Migratory arthritic pains

_____ Muscle spasms/twitches

_____ Feeling spacey

_____Violent temper

_____Arthritic-like pain

_____Anxiety

_____Allergies

_____Constipation/diarrhea

_____Abdominal gas/bloating

_____Weight gain

_____Weight loss

_____Fatigue

_____Drowsiness

_____Puffy hands/feet

_____PMS

_____Panic attacks

_____Hatband headache

_____Thinning eyebrows

_____Cold hands/feet

_____Subnormal temperature

_____Unmotivated/can't cope

_____Insomnia

_____Trouble waking

_____Gas that feels "stuck"

_____Incomplete BM

_____Pain in lower abdomen

_____Pain in upper abdomen

_____Ravenous hunger

_____Symptoms worse at night

_____Swollen sore breasts

_____Night sweats

_____Depression

_____Melancholy

Add up the numbers and enter your total here: _____

The many and varied symptoms you may be experiencing have everything to do with what you put into your body, whether it's food, air, or water. A score of 50 or more shows that your filtering organs are not functioning at their optimal level. They need some time to cleanse and rebalance. Removing the foods and chemicals that are causing the problems is the first step in detoxing.

Intolerance, Allergies, and Sensitivities

You can be sensitive to a food or chemical, but not necessarily allergic. Your body can also exhibit an intolerance to something and yet not suffer an allergic reaction. These intolerances and sensitivities come from your liver's inability to break down chemicals and proteins in the detoxification pathways.

Food sensitivities can happen because most people don't chew their food to liquid. Remember, digestion begins in the mouth. While your teeth masticate food, digestive enzymes are released in your saliva. As a result of not chewing properly, your food is not completely broken down and enters your intestines as particles that can get absorbed into the bloodstream. This creates antigen-antibody or allergic reactions. These allergy complexes can travel anywhere in the body—to the joints to cause arthritis symptoms, to the brain to trigger headaches, to the nasal passages to cause sinus reactions, to the intestines to create an irritable bowel, and to the skin to trigger eczema. Your stomach is not designed to have to break down large pieces of meat, fries, or pizza dough. Chew your food well and avoid indigestion!

Healthy Tidbits

It can be difficult to determine food sensitivities because one can have a reaction anywhere from one hour to three days after ingesting the food. There are special blood tests (called IgG testing) you can have done that will tell you what foods you are sensitive to. Ask your health-care professional.

Allergy Self-Test

There are blood tests available to determine if you have an allergy to a food or not. If you suspect you have an allergy, you can try this self-test recommended by Sandra Cabot, M.D., then later confirm it with your doctor.

Just before eating a meal, sit quietly in a relaxed state. Place your fingers on your wrist pulse and measure the beats per minute, normally 55 to 75 beats. Once this is established, eat the food you are sensitive to, making sure to chew well. After 20 minutes, take your pulse rate again. If it has increased by more than 10 beats per minute, you may be intolerant of the food. If you experience symptoms of dizziness, nausea, or discomfort, you will want to eliminate this food from your diet during the five-week detox program and see if your health improves.

Substituting One Food for Another

There are certain foods that commonly cause *food allergies.* These are first considered when people suffer from symptoms of *food intolerance.* The detox program takes you off some of these foods and offers excellent substitutes that you will want to include in your diet long after the detox is over.

def•i•ni•tion

A **food allergy** is how your body's immune system reacts to a food, typically small particles that have entered the bloodstream, when it sees the food as a foreign invader. **Food intolerance** is when your digestive system has an adverse reaction to a food or food ingredient.

The following table lists the top 10 foods you may be sensitive to and not even know it, along with some healthy substitutes.

Food Allergy	Substitute
Eggs	Whole grains, turkey, chicken
Cow's milk	Goat, nut, rice, and coconut milk
Fish	Beans, legumes, chicken
Shellfish	Chicken, meat, beans, nuts, seeds
Wheat	Rice, quinoa, amaranth, millet

Gluten	Rice, quinoa, amaranth, millet
Chocolate	Carob, sesame halva
Peanuts	Pumpkin and sunflower seeds, nuts
Tree nuts	Pumpkin, sunflower, and sesame seeds
Soy	Fruits, vegetables, legumes, nuts

You may think that just avoiding the food will prevent you from ingesting it. That's wishful thinking. Wheat, eggs, and milk are used in many commercial products; peanuts may have been processed in equipment that was then used for another food; and soy is a bulking agent for hamburgers, baked goods, and many processed items. In Chapter 2, you will learn how genetically modified foods contain the genes of a food you may be allergic to. All the more important in surviving the labyrinth of food contamination, you should eat foods in their natural, unprocessed form, from farms and gardens that you know provide the highest-quality organic foods. (I'll tell you all about buying and eating organic foods in Chapter 5.)

The Actual Benefits

As a result of doing the five-week detox program, the majority of people report feelings of extreme well-being. They look and feel lighter and healthier; they have more energy and can remember where they left their car keys, meaning improved memory.

Detoxification of your organs and cleansing your bloodstream enhances your body's ability to digest food and absorb the necessary vitamins and minerals. Getting the nutrients that nature intended will result in some surprising benefits, including looking years younger, improved sex drive, and better sleep.

Sleep Better

I once had a young fashion editor in a detox program who complained of severe insomnia. Once she began to detoxify, she complained that she was sleeping too much. Go figure. When was the last time you had a full night of restful sleep? This is the most important function your body should complete. It is during sleep that your organs and tissues grow and repair. Presently your body runs on stimulants: sugar, caffeine, alcohol, and tobacco. Once you remove them from your diet, your body can relax and experience some deep REM sleep.

Look Younger

Just getting enough sleep can take years off your face. However, it is not uncommon when detoxifying to be accosted by your friends and co-workers, demanding to know why you look so good. You can tell them that it is because you are no longer bloated in the face and your big round belly has subsided enough to button your favorite pants again. You might mention that you feel crazy like a kid and are thinking of starting tango classes. Or you can say you've been taking better care of yourself by detoxifying your organs and eating only the highest-quality foods.

Boost Your Immune System

Having a strong immune system is a way of knowing your body's security system is turned on and defending the home front. When working properly, your immune system attacks any foreign antigens and rids them from the body. When overwhelmed, weakened, or destroyed, it can attack its own cells, which is the case with autoimmune diseases, such as the following:

- Multiple sclerosis
- Systemic lupus erythematosis
- Rheumatoid arthritis
- Graves' disease
- Hashimoto's thyroiditis

Detoxifying your body can go a long way in helping to strengthen your immune system. By cleansing the blood and lymph tissues your immunity increases, the system grows stronger, and your health improves.

Lose Weight

Weight gain is a symptom of a sluggish liver due to overeating refined, processed food. I suggest you focus on eating the proper foods and forget about your weight for now. Even in the two-week pre-detox, when eating the highest-quality organic grains, vegetables, fruits, and animal protein, your metabolism will change and you should lose weight. Watch what happens when you begin to "eat to live" rather than "live to eat." Refrain from getting on the scale for a while and just enjoy the way your clothes begin to fit much looser.

That Certain Something

I can't tell you exactly when you will feel it. For me it's about halfway through the detox program. Suddenly there comes a point when you feel fantastic. After a detox one of my students told me, "I never believed I could feel this good. I want to have this feeling all the time." It's not something you can put into words, but suffice it to say, your outlook on life improves, your moods are lighter, and you handle stress in a more optimistic way. Your newly cleansed liver helps keep your temper under wraps, and irritability is a thing of the past. Not bad, not bad at all!

The wonderful thing that happens after detoxing is you want to continue feeling good and looking good while maintaining a high energy level. You've gotten to a nice place with your health, but there's more to discover. As you follow the recommended eating plans suggested in Chapters 9 through 13, keep in mind that they are also the perfect lifestyle change to keep you fit and healthy.

The Least You Need to Know

- Regular detoxification helps you sleep better, look younger, and strengthens your immune system.

- Drugs, hormones, and heavy metals can build up in your system over time and need to be detoxified properly.

- Chronic fatigue syndrome, fibromyalgia, and multiple chemical sensitivities are related to your body's inability to naturally detoxify.

- Always consult your doctor before undertaking a detoxification program on your own.

- The Lifestyle, Sensitivities, and Symptoms questionnaires are excellent guidelines for determining your need to detoxify.

- Food sensitivities can be alleviated by eliminating the suspect food for a period of time, or substituting a different food.

Chapter 2

What There Is to Detox

In This Chapter

- ◆ What's in and on the food we eat
- ◆ Dangers of pesticides and herbicides
- ◆ Food additives
- ◆ Toxic air pollutants
- ◆ What's in your drinking water
- ◆ The truth about artificial sweeteners

Having completed the questionnaires in Chapter 1, you realize you probably have a few things to detox from your body. Concerned about your health, maybe you would like to lose a few pounds and give this detox thing a go but you're not quite sure what toxins you're dealing with. It is hard to imagine what chemicals might be floating around in your bloodstream when you can't see or smell anything remotely like a chemical.

In this chapter, you will find out what specific toxins and chemicals you are dealing with—just because you can't see the chemicals, doesn't mean they aren't there.

Your Chemical Cocktails

If you are like most people, you begin your morning with a cup of tea or coffee and a dose of DDT, malathion, paraquat, diazinon, and a bit of Round-up (sprayed on the coffee bean). Milk or cream comes with acceptable amounts of bovine growth hormone, a shot of antibiotics, and a few steroid molecules for good measure. One or two teaspoons of sugar filtered through slaughtered bone ash lets the grains spill into your cup without caking. A bowl of genetically modified cornflakes carries up to 50 different pesticides just to bring it to your table on this lovely morning. You reach for a sip of orange juice that required 253 gallons of water and half a gallon of tractor fuel before landing on your table. Good morning, America, your daily chemical intake has only just begun.

Pesticides

A pesticide is a poisonous chemical sprayed on your food in order to eradicate any insect, creature, bacteria, mold, microbe, weed, bird, fish, mollusk … you get the picture. The problem is, many of those pesticides are deadly for humans as well. Sure, they are designed to kill pests—but they will eventually kill other animals, including the person applying the chemicals to the plants.

> **Detox Alert**
>
> Apiarists (beekeepers) around the globe are seriously concerned over rapidly waning honeybee populations. Theories as to what is causing the decline include cell phone radiation, pesticides, mites, global warming, and genetically modified crops, but nothing specific has been proven.

> **Pure Insights**
>
> Without bees to pollinate our crops, humans will have only four years of life left.
> —Albert Einstein

As defined by the Environmental Protection Agency (EPA), ecological risk assessment is a process whereby toxicity and exposure estimates are evaluated to see if wildlife, plants, and humans are subject to harm from the intended use of a pesticide. All pesticides pose some risk, and environmental concentration estimates are critical in estimating ecological risk.

Through observation and research we now know that there are 70,000 synthetic chemicals used in our environment. The chemical industry admits at least 50 of these synthetic industrial chemicals are seriously toxic to plant, animal, and human life, with more being discovered every day. In 1996, *Science* magazine published a study showing how when two or more nontoxic chemicals are combined in the environment, they become 1,600 times as powerful as they would be on their own. These combinations can have a major long-range impact on the health of fetal development and small children. As to the effects on adults, with two out of three Americans developing cancer, I feel safe suggesting you should reduce your exposure to these chemicals whenever possible.

Washing your produce may reduce some surface chemicals, but not all of them. Plus, many of these foods are sprayed from a young stage, so they have the pesticides as part of their inner fiber. You can use a produce detergent, which is made to break down these petroleum-based chemicals, or you can buy organic, chemical-free produce.

Detox Alert

Pesticides are also used in homes, schools, parks, hospitals, and office buildings. According to the National Resources Defense Council, 74 percent of American households (70 million) used some type of pesticide at a cost of $1.9 million in 1994.

If you cannot find organic produce, the good news is that you can lower your pesticide exposure by almost 90 percent by avoiding the top 12 most contaminated fruits and vegetables and eating the least contaminated instead. The top 12 produce ranking was developed by analysts at the not-for-profit Environmental Working Group (EWG), based on the results of nearly 43,000 tests for pesticides on produce collected by the U.S. Department of Agriculture and the U.S. Food and Drug Administration between 2000 and 2004.

According to this analysis, eating the 12 most contaminated fruits and vegetables will expose a person to about 15 pesticides per day, on average. Eating the 12 least contaminated will expose a person to less than 2 pesticides per day. It's a place to begin.

Here are the fruits and vegetables that have the highest amounts of pesticides sprayed on them:

1. Peaches
2. Apples
3. Sweet bell peppers
4. Celery
5. Nectarines
6. Strawberries
7. Cherries
8. Pears
9. Grapes (imported)
10. Spinach
11. Lettuce
12. Potatoes

The least amounts of pesticides are sprayed on the following:

1. Onions
2. Avocado
3. Sweet corn (frozen)
4. Pineapples
5. Mango
6. Asparagus
7. Sweet peas (frozen)
8. Kiwi fruit
9. Bananas
10. Cabbage
11. Broccoli
12. Papaya

Until you have the items memorized, keep the list with you when you go shopping. This way you can refer to it when there are no organic options. You can also speak to the supermarket manager and let him or her know that you are willing to buy organic products if the store will carry them. The stores will stock organic foods if you, the consumer, will buy them. Money always talks.

Herbicides

Herbicides are right up there with pesticides in the deadly poison category. They are designed to kill other plants, weeds in particular. What some people consider a weed, such as the magnificent dandelion, others honor for its high nutrient content and healing properties. Herbicides target a plant's specific hormones in order to destroy it without harming the protected crop. It is interesting to note that herbicides have been found to disrupt the endocrine (hormone) systems of animals with the suspicion that they are endocrine disruptors for humans as well. (More about that in a moment.)

def•i•ni•tion

Atrazine is a widely used herbicide that the Environmental Protection Agency believes can possibly cause harm to endangered wildlife. Banned in Europe but sprayed heavily on corn, sugar, and other crops in America, 60 million pounds of atrazine make their way into rivers, lakes, streams, and drinking water supplies annually.

The National Resources Defense Council (www. nrdc.org) reports that in 1996, an estimated 36 million pounds of herbicides, including *atrazine*, were applied to 99 percent of harvested corn acreage in Iowa. This is food grown in Iowa and used in food products and as animal feed across the country.

An estimated 10.8 million pounds of herbicides were applied to almost 100 percent of soybean acreage that same year. In addition, 1.8 million pounds of insecticides were applied to 17 percent of Iowa corn acreage. Because of this, 24 different herbicides were found to be contaminating 95 percent of Iowa's drinking water.

Endocrine Disrupters

Your endocrine glands make chemicals called hormones and pass them straight into the bloodstream. Hormones communicate with the body and bring about changes in your physical growth, metabolism, cellular repair, sexual reproduction, digestion, and internal balance. Environmental chemicals disrupt the intricate network that regulates your body's reproductive system, your ovaries and testes, as well as your pituitary, thyroid, adrenal, and thymus glands. They are sprayed on your food and served with a nice dose of artificial flavorings and colorings.

These synthetic chemicals actually alter the way your body produces hormones, and this in turn affects the functions those hormones would normally be taking care of easily. The endocrine disrupting chemicals I am referring to are as follows:

- ◆ Dioxin
- ◆ PCBs
- ◆ DDT
- ◆ Pesticides

- ◆ Herbicides
- ◆ Plasticizers
- ◆ Diethylstilbestrol (DES)

In today's environment you will run smack dab into these bad boys every time you ingest contaminated water, food, and/or air. They also leach out of plastic bottles, plastic containers, or plastic wrap and accumulate in your fatty tissue. By watching how they affect other vertebrate animals in nature, scientists have drawn the conclusion that these chemicals are disrupting our endocrine system also.

Now, are you still wondering what there is in your body that needs detoxing? If so, keep reading.

GMOs (Genetically Modified Organisms)

When genetically modified organisms (GMOs) first became big news in the 1990s, it seemed like something out of a science-fiction movie. Crossing the gene pool of one plant or animal with another or genes from an animal with a plant seemed too out there for most people. Believe me, it still is way out there and in the ensuing years has disrupted the lives of farmers, consumers, and the whole agricultural industry.

The irony of genetic engineering is that even as we protest the inclusion of foreign genes into our food supply, athletes are injecting genes into their bodies, hoping for an edge over their competitors as they strive for more endurance, speed, and strength. Gene therapy for disease is the hope for the future, allowing us to live long, healthy lives free from disease. It looks like the bionic woman may be but a generation or two away.

Healthy Tidbits

Genetic engineering allows a company to own the patent on a particular plant by modifying the genes in the seeds. No one knows for certain if biotechnology is safe or better than how we currently grow our food. The biggest concern is that a small group of companies could control the world's food supply.

The Food Additives You Love

The introduction of chemicals, preservatives, and colorings to our food supply has changed the way we eat. The sole purpose of these additives is to disguise the fact that in the processing of foods, taste and color are lost, along with the vital nutrients your body needs to stay healthy. Appealing colors and flavorings say "fresh" to the consumer. Brown food is not as appetizing.

Food additives have been used in the production of processed food for quite some time. Because the color, texture, and nutrient content of a food are altered when processed, they need to be added back, but in synthetic form. These food additives—preservatives, emulsifiers, glazing agents, artificial colorings, artificial flavorings, and taste enhancers—are known to cause allergic reactions in children and adults.

When reading food labels, you will want to avoid these food additives whenever possible:

- Food colorings
- Preservatives: sorbates, benzoates, sulfites, nitrates, nitrites, propionates
- Synthetic antioxidants: gallates, TBHQ, BHA, BHT
- Flavor enhancers: monosodium glutamate (MSG), ribonucleotides, hydrolyzed vegetable protein
- Artificial flavors
- Aspartame

- ◆ Caffeine

- ◆ Saccharin

- ◆ Sulfites

Food labels don't always list the exact ingredients. For example, monosodium glutamate (MSG) can be included in the term "spices." MSG is manufactured/ processed free glutamic acid, not found in organic, unprocessed meat, poultry, fish, or vegetables. If you are sensitive to MSG, remember this when reading food labels. MSG-sensitive people may experience headaches, sinus blockage, lightheadedness, or heart palpitations when consuming food containing MSG.

Food additives allow for longer shelf life and cheaper ingredient costs. This in turn increases a food manufacturer's profits. The majority of additives tested are safe, but many have not been adequately tested and there are many that are harmful to your health. Read labels carefully so you can avoid these chemicals.

Bovine Growth Hormone

Dairy cows are injected with genetically engineered bovine growth hormone, iBGH, to increase production of milk. It was soon discovered that this process creates severe inflammation in the cow's udder called mastitis. This leads to high amounts of infected pus in the milk. To counter this, a more-than-usual allotment of antibiotics is fed to dairy cows, and residues of these antibiotics shows up in the drinking milk.

Another distressing side effect of injecting growth hormone into cows is elevation of Insulin-like Growth Factor (IGF-1) in people who drink the milk. When women drink milk laced with IGF-1 there is an increased incidence of breast cancer. The end result is a food product that is nearly impossible for human beings to digest and one that, after careful engineering, can be linked to cancer.

The Most Common Preservatives

It is almost impossible to avoid chemical preservatives unless you grow all your own food organically and prepare all your meals from scratch. Added for food safety during long transports and the extended shelf life of many products, preservatives are a necessary part of our food culture. Otherwise, commercial bread would get moldy, oils would go rancid, and packaged meals would spoil.

A few commonly used preservatives are: calcium propionate, *nitrates*, disodium EDTA, and BHA. Even dried fruit, potato chips, and trail mix contain sulfur-based preservatives. Regulations require preservatives to be food grade and quantity must not exceed what is needed to preserve an item.

def•i•ni•tion

> **Nitrates** are used in combination with salt to inhibit bacterial growth in meats and for flavoring and color fixing in red meat, poultry, and fish products. Nitrite salts can react with certain amines (derivatives of ammonia) in food to produce nitrosamines, many of which are known to cause cancer.

Salt and sugar are natural preservatives used in older times and are still used in many canned and processed foods today.

The Air You Breathe

Particles and gases in the air you breathe are known as air pollution. That gray smog suspended over a city is the gas ozone, a major pollutant in the warming of our atmosphere. It can come from car, truck, and industry emissions and large dairy factories emitting volatile organic compounds into the atmosphere.

According to the EPA, air pollution can come from many different sources, including factories, power plants, dry cleaners, cars, buses, trucks, and even windblown dust and wildfires. Air pollution can threaten the health of human beings, animals, trees, lakes, and crops, as well as damage the ozone layer and buildings. Air pollution can also cause haze, reducing visibility in national parks and wilderness areas.

Air pollution can be responsible for asthma in children and the elderly, allergies, bronchitis, and lung cancer. In a study by scientists at the University of Southern California, children who lived within 1,600 feet of a major highway exhaled 3 percent less air at a 7 percent slower rate than children living a mile away. The concern is that these children will develop smaller lungs and therefore have a higher risk of lung cancer and other infections.

Under the Clean Air Act, the EPA sets limits on how much of a pollutant is allowed in the air anywhere in the United States. Although national air quality has improved over the last 20 years, many challenges remain in protecting public health and the environment. On the EPA's website (www.epa.gov), you can view and track the levels of pollutants in the air and which sources they are coming from. This can be a great help to asthma sufferers, the elderly, and those with respiratory issues.

What Dissolves in Your Water

Next to food and air, water is the most important ingredient we need to survive. Much of the water that covers our Earth is unfit for us to drink. Ocean water is too salty to drink, lakes and rivers are contaminated with agriculture run-off and treated sewage, leaching toxins into soil contaminates well water, rain water contains chemical impurities, and mountain streams are infected with Giardia.

Chemicals, toxins, and organisms make their way into our water supply in minute quantities that can have an accumulative effect in our bodies. Then humans go and add chemicals to the water for the sake of good health. Go figure.

The Fluoride Controversy

Fluoride is best known as the chemical added to drinking water and toothpaste to prevent dental decay. The fluoride in your water is made up of industrial waste products from the phosphate fertilizer industry.

According to Dr. Paul Connett of the Fluoride Action Network, fluoride has minimal benefit when swallowed. Any benefits that accrue from the use of fluoride come from the direct application of fluoride to the outside of teeth and not from ingestion. There is no need to expose all other tissues to fluoride by swallowing it.

> **Pure Insights**
>
> Fluoride is a pharmacologically very active compound with an action on a variety of enzymes and tissues in the body already in low concentrations. In concentrations not far above those recommended it has overt toxic actions. I am quite convinced that water fluoridation, in a not-too-distant future, will be consigned to medical history.
> —Dr. Arvid Carlsson, winner of the Nobel Prize for Medicine (2000)

The National Research Council (NRC) states that drinking fluoridated water can cause dementia in adults and low IQ in children. It also creates thyroid problems, diminished bone strength, and bone cancer in males under 20 years old.

As a matter of fact, the American Dental Association has advised parents that fluoridated water should not be given to babies. This can cause dental fluorosis, a permanent tooth defect. Early life exposures may also damage the brain, causing learning deficits and other problems.

Is Chlorine Worth the Risk?

The purpose of adding chlorine to our water is to disinfect it and prevent contamination from microorganisms. This it does well, but chlorine also has its dark side. It can change your good HDL into the bad LDL that clogs your arteries. Based on a study in which chlorine was fed to a test group of chickens, Dr. Joseph Price, author of *Coronaries/Cholesterol/Chlorine*, concluded that nothing can negate the incontrovertible fact that the basic cause of atherosclerosis and resulting entities such as heart attacks and stroke is chlorine.

Also, drinking chlorinated water has been officially linked to an increased incidence of bladder and colon cancer. According to a study published in the *Journal of the National Cancer Institute*, long-term drinking of chlorinated water appears to increase a person's risk of developing bladder cancer as much as 80 percent.

And if that's not enough to keep you from swallowing the pool water, consider that a study carried out in Hartford, Connecticut, the first of its kind in North America, found that "women with breast cancer have 50 to 60 percent higher levels of organochlorines (chlorination byproducts) in their breast tissue than women without breast cancer."

> **Pure Insights**
>
> Drinking tap water that is chlorinated is hazardous if not deadly to your health.
>
> —Dr. Martin Fox, *Healthy Water for Longer Life*

Your best bet is to install a reliable water filtration system in your home, or at least your kitchen sink. There are many on the market, but your choices consist of carbon filtration, reverse osmosis, distillation, and ozone treatment.

Flushed Away

Ever wonder where all the pharmaceutical drugs go that you ingest and then urinate out through your bladder? The EPA has found drugs and personal care products are literally being flushed from sewage treatment plants into rivers or are leaching into groundwater from septic systems. In a 1999 EPA survey of 139 streams around the country, 80 percent of the samples contained residues of drugs like painkillers, blood pressure medicine, hormones, and antibiotics.

This is also being seen in other countries around the world as more and more people take medication or discard outdated medicines down the drain. With water becoming a precious commodity, more communities are returning treated sewage back into their water supplies and low levels of these contaminants are making it through the treatment process and into the drinking water. At this point nobody can really say what the effects on our health will be, but it doesn't take much to ascertain that all those chemicals, combined in a glass of water, can be one very toxic cocktail.

Artificial Sweeteners

Despite repeated warnings from the scientific community that artificial sweeteners can debilitate your health, people continue to consume them in soft drinks, toothpaste, desserts, medications, dietetic canned foods, and numerous other packaged foods.

Aspartame, the main ingredient in NutraSweet and Equal, can now be found in thousands of products and is the focus of thousands of consumer complaints to the FDA for health-related problems. The EPA recommends that you limit your consumption of aspartame to 7.8 milligrams a day. A 1-liter (approximately 1 quart) aspartame-sweetened beverage contains about 56 milligrams of methanol. Heavy users of aspartame-containing products consume as much as 250 milligrams of methanol daily, or 32 times the EPA limit. The nonprofit, informational website www.dorway.com/symptoms.html is dedicated to showing the health dangers of aspartame and removing it from our food and beverages. There you will find a list of 92 health symptoms believed to be caused by eating foods containing aspartame. Symptoms include the following:

- Headaches
- Rashes
- Seizures
- Depression
- Gastrointestinal symptoms

- Memory loss
- Blurred vision
- Slurred speech
- Neurological disorders

What makes it so deadly to the body is that 10 percent of aspartame is made up of methanol/wood alcohol, which is a deadly poison. Methanol breaks down into formic acid and formaldehyde in the body. Formaldehyde is a deadly neurotoxin known to destroy brain cells.

An EPA assessment of methanol states that it "is considered a cumulative poison due to the low rate of excretion once it is absorbed. In the body, methanol is oxidized to formaldehyde and formic acid; both of these metabolites are toxic."

Pure Insights

If we support technology that destroys nature, the destruction of nature leads to our destruction, all species, but particularly our destruction. If everybody has cancer, if children are developing cancer at the age of 5 and 10 years old, there's no sense to anything. Nothing takes precedence over us staying healthy and us staying alive, of keeping the earth alive, keeping the Mother alive.

—Dr. Wally Burnstein, D.O.

The next generation of artificial sweeteners brings us sucralose, which is sold under the name Splenda. A high-intensity sugar substitute, Splenda is noncaloric and about 600 times sweeter than sucrose (white table sugar). The chemical process to make sucralose alters the chemical composition of the sugar so much that it is somehow converted to a fructo-galactose molecule. This type of sugar molecule does not occur in nature and therefore your body does not possess the ability to properly metabolize it. Few human studies of safety have been published on sucralose, and it is to be avoided on your detox program and lifestyle eating plan.

Your five-week detox program calls for the total elimination of artificial sweeteners from your diet. You can substitute natural sweeteners like raw, unrefined honey; maple syrup; brown rice syrup; stevia; and xylitol during certain weeks, for your baking and cooking needs.

The Least You Need to Know

- Pesticides and herbicides are known to be toxic to people, animals, and plants.

- Herbicides have been found to disrupt the endocrine (hormone) systems of animals; they may well have the same effect on humans.

- The sole purpose of food additives is to disguise the fact that good taste and appealing color are lacking.

- When you inhale heavy metal particles from air pollution, they enter your lungs and from there get into your blood stream and organs.

- A major downside to the prolific use of pharmaceutical drugs by a growing population is that they eventually end up in your drinking water.

- What makes aspartame so deadly to the body is that 10 percent of the synthetic sweetener is made up of methanol/wood alcohol, which is a deadly poison.

You Are What You Eat

In This Chapter

- ◆ The sad state of the Standard American Diet

- ◆ The top 10 worst foods you can eat

- ◆ Why some other foods are not good for you

- ◆ Lack of fiber = constipation

- ◆ Overcoming your addictions

- ◆ Exploring new foods and tastes

Americans consume over 1 billion pounds—and 1 trillion calories—of food each day. To feed a country of nearly 300 million people, our agricultural system consumes enormous quantities of fuel, fertilizers, water, and pesticides, and sets aside enormous tracts of land just for feeding the livestock Americans consume! Ultimately, a diet rich in fatty animal products and poor in whole grains, fruits, and vegetables consumes the consumer.

In this chapter, you will learn how eating a diet based on processed foods leads to high rates of heart disease, stroke, certain cancers, diabetes, and obesity. These common diseases cause millions of premature deaths each year.

Your SAD Diet

Ironically, the acronym for the Standard American Diet is SAD. It pretty much sums up our fast-food lifestyle in three letters. This translates to mean a processed and health-degenerating series of meals consumed more for entertainment than for nutrient value. The SAD diet is high in saturated animal fats and refined carbohydrates, possibly fried and/or covered with lots of cheese, or containing large amounts of sugar. These foods are low in fiber and are difficult to eliminate from the bowels. Thus, you are what you *don't* eliminate. This can also cause serious cellulite to form on your thighs and buttocks, but that is the least of your worries.

When you are involved in various day-to-day crises, it is difficult to see that your body is breaking down under the strain. With too much to do and not enough time, we run from one thing to another, grabbing a quick bite to eat along the way. Those fast-food burgers, fries, and milkshakes put stress on your organs by causing an acid condition to build up in your blood. A high acid blood pH can lead to degeneration and disease. The Standard American Diet creates an acid condition because the foods eaten are all acid-forming foods.

In a nutshell, the Standard American Diet = external stress + acid-forming foods = internal stress + acid blood pH = disease.

Healthy Tidbits _____

Health pioneer Herbert M. Shelton was fond of pointing out how people and their doctors are totally ignorant about the origin of disease. At his spa in San Antonio, Texas, back in the '30s he railed against the Standard American Diet and prescribed a diet high in alkaline-forming foods (fruits and vegetables), food combining, and periodic fasting to safely rid the intestines of putrefied and toxic foods. Shelton lived a long and healthy life helping people detoxify their bodies until he died at the age of 89.

When you take time to detoxify, you give your physical body a break from the stress-causing foods that you eat every day. You probably learned about these foods the hard way, by having a bad reaction. For others of you these foods can be the cause of your physical suffering, and once you are off of them, some of that suffering will ease up.

Here are the six major food culprits that create internal organ stress:

◆ Refined wheat flour: cakes, cookies, pasta, and bread

◆ Pasteurized dairy: milk, cheese, and yogurt

◆ Refined sugar: in all forms

◆ Caffeine: coffee, chocolate, tea, and soda pop

◆ Alcohol: beer, wine, and hard liquor

◆ Artificial sweeteners and flavor enhancers

These nutrient-deficient foods can clog your major filtering organs, weaken your immune system, and contribute to the overgrowth of yeast and parasites in your body. This is why we eliminate them for detoxing purposes.

Fast Food for Fast Times

We are presently in the fifth generation of people eating a refined food diet. The mounting evidence reveals health problems with anxiety, obesity, hypoglycemia, diabetes, autoimmune disease, and an overgrowth of Candida albicans topping the list. In other words, fast foods can quickly make you sick.

Pure Insights

In 1970, Americans spent about $6 billion on fast food; in 2000, they spent more than $110 billion dollars. Americans now spend more money on fast food than on higher education, personal computers, computer software, or new cars. They spend more on fast food than on movies, books, magazines, newspapers, videos, and recorded music—combined.

—Eric Schlosser, *Fast Food Nation*

The 10 worst foods for you listed in health books, on Internet health sites, and condemned by nutritionists are more than likely a part of your daily diet:

1. French fries
2. Donuts
3. Potato and corn chips
4. Soda pop
5. Snack cakes
6. Candy and granola bars
7. Fast-food burgers
8. Fat-free cookies
9. Bagels
10. Pretzels

I would throw into the mix pizza, ice cream, cheese, bacon, and those fancy coffee drinks that cost a fortune. Not a fruit or vegetable on the list. The french fry at 200 calories of toxic saturated fat per serving is not a food, it is a health hazard.

Stress-Causing Foods

You'll be eliminating stress-causing foods from your diet during your detox program—no need to worry about what you'll eat in their place. In Chapters 9 through 13, you will find everything you need, from instructions to shopping lists, to help you make the transition smooth and easy. For every food you eliminate there will be something equally as delicious to replace it.

Let's take a look at what you will be giving up during the detox program. Perhaps once you understand how bad these foods can be for you it will make getting rid of them easier.

Milk, Cheese, and Yogurt

Consider that you are what you eat and what you don't eliminate. Now imagine a large animal standing out in a field chewing cud. You eat and drink large quantities of milk, cheese, and yogurt from this animal. It is a powerful food designed by Mother Nature to strengthen a baby calf's body as quickly as possible to keep up with the herd and avoid predators. On the other hand, human mother's milk is designed to feed the baby's brain first, while slowly growing the body. Humans are the only species who drink milk into adulthood. Milk is for babies and mother's milk is always the best.

def•i•ni•tion

Lactose intolerance is the body's inability to digest the sugars in cow's milk once the milk has been pasteurized. People who get tested for lactose intolerance and find they are *not* sensitive to lactose, but know they cannot tolerate milk products, may be sensitive to casein, a protein found in milk.

Milk must be pasteurized and homogenized before being sold. This renders the food indigestible because humans lack the enzyme to break down the sugar in cow's milk. Naturally, the intention to protect you from becoming infected with salmonella and E. coli was a good one. However, the resulting *lactose intolerance* can affect your health in a number of ways:

- Allergic reaction causing bloating, gas, indigestion

- Repeated infections of the ears, lungs, and sinuses

- Overabundance of mucus

- Asthma

- Irritable bowel syndrome

- Aggravation of autoimmune diseases

- Formation of cysts and lumps in thyroid and breasts

Also remember from Chapter 2 how cows are fed excessive amounts of antibiotics and injected with bovine growth hormones. These poisons leave a measurable amount of residue in the milk, resulting in a highly toxic food product.

Consider how much dairy you eat on a daily basis:

- In the morning do you have milk, cream, or half and half with your coffee, tea, or cereal?

- Do you have yogurt with fruit and nuts for a snack?

- For lunch is there cheese on your sandwich and milk again in your coffee?

- Does your afternoon snack include cheese, yogurt, or milk?

- Does dinner include a cream sauce on your pasta or chicken?

- How often do you have ice cream for dessert or a snack?

> **Healthy Tidbits**
>
> If you are not sure how much dairy you eat or you're having a moment of dairy denial, take a few days and write down what you eat and drink at each meal and snack. Eating a fast-food diet means eating fast and not even noticing what and how much you are consuming. Keeping a journal can be a real eye-opener.

Martha called me, distraught because her 16-year-old son had horrible acne and was constantly fatigued. She brought Jason to see me and I put them both on a five-week detox program. Martha was overweight and unable to sleep. She saw this as a great opportunity to help herself and Jason at the same time. After two weeks of being away from pizza, milkshakes, and ice cream, Jason's skin cleared up. Following his detox he went out for a slice with his buddies and the next day his skin broke out again. He now knew what triggered the acne and gave up pizza for good.

The fact is, dairy products create an overabundance of mucus if you have weak digestion. Because today's milk supply is pasteurized, homogenized, and loaded with chemicals, even if you have a strong digestive system, you can be adversely affected by including it in your diet. A mucus-forming diet of wheat flour, sugar, meat, dairy, and fat can cause weakness and weight gain. The only way to rebuild and strengthen your body is to detoxify and then avoid these stress foods.

Dr. Joseph Mercola, M.D., recommends that for your children to get their daily calcium allowance, they need to do the following:

◆ Get equal amounts of calcium and magnesium in the form of foods rich in these minerals, high-quality supplements, or goat's milk.

◆ Get vitamin D in the form of sun exposure in the summer and cod liver oil in the winter.

◆ Drink water instead of soda pop or fruit juice.

◆ Eat enough high-quality protein for optimal bone density.

Although still controversial in many states, more and more people are buying raw, unpasteurized, nonhomogenized, grass-fed organic cow's milk from small dairy farms in their areas. Consumers have also turned to drinking organic milk, which is still pasteurized and not always from grass-fed cows. Since there are so many alternatives to drinking cow's milk, why not explore those first?

Wheat, the Glue That Binds

There are many types of grains, but in North America we tend to eat mostly wheat that has been highly refined. Refining strips the grain of its living wheat germ, bran, and most of its nutrients. Once reduced to white flour, it is fit only for making glue. The food industry then adds back synthetic nutrients and labels the product "enriched." Seems like a lot of work just to come back to where they started.

The main staple in the Standard American Diet is this white enriched flour. Breakfast for many Americans includes a muffin, bagel, or toast with coffee, milk, and sugar. Lunch is often a sandwich on refined white bread. Snacks might consist of cookies, chips, or hard-baked pretzels. Dinner can include table rolls, pizza, pasta, or crusty white bread. Consuming this amount of wheat every day can set you up to develop food sensitivities or allergies.

This can be a disconcerting moment if wheat flour is a primary food source for you. Fortunately in today's health-food markets there are a wide variety of delicious breads made with whole grain flour such as *spelt*, Kamut, brown rice, millet, and rye. These breads are delicious. You will also find sprouted grain breads that are so rich with nutrients that you only need a small slice to feel satisfied. Try several different kinds of breads until you find one that you like. They are perfect toasted with a spread of almond butter and fruit jam. Or use them to make your favorite sandwich. This is not a detox program of deprivation, but rather a journey to discover new ways to achieve optimal health.

def•i•ni•tion

Spelt is a nutritious whole grain thought to be one of the first grains used to make bread. A distant cousin to wheat, spelt dates back some 7,000 years and is mentioned in the Bible. It has a delicious nutlike flavor and does not seem to cause digestive sensitivities in people intolerant to wheat.

Suffering with Constipation

Constipation can be the result of eating a SAD diet. This is due to a lack of fiber in your diet. With no fiber to help the colon generate peristaltic action, it becomes lazy and sluggish, clogged and backed up, leading your system to literally poison itself. This can lead to a variety of intestinal diseases such as colon cancer, diverticulosis, diverticulitis, irritable bowel syndrome, and colitis. All of this can be prevented by eating quality fiber from whole, unrefined foods. Also taking the probiotics acidophilus and bifidus along with certain fermented foods goes a long way in keeping your bowels healthy. (See Chapter 6 for more on probiotics.)

Some schools of thought say after every meal you should have a bowel movement. Some say twice a day and others suggest once in the morning. The important thing to notice is that they all mention that you evacuate your bowels daily, not every other day and especially not once a week. Your digestive system is designed to discharge all waste matter, the sooner the better. Not to worry. During the detox program you will be eating a high-fiber diet, allowing you to eliminate a whole lot of waste you didn't even know was there. Your energy will increase, your moods will lighten, and your weight will begin to regulate itself.

Overcoming Addictions

For purposes of the detox program I will define addiction as being in a state of psychological and/or physiological dependence on any one of the following:

◆ Drugs: pharmaceutical and recreational

◆ Food: sweet desserts, salty snacks, chocolate

- ◆ Caffeine: coffee, soda pop, energy drinks

- ◆ Alcohol: wine, beer, hard liquor

- ◆ Cigarettes: regular or light, organic or nonorganic

Every one of these items is standard fare for most of the world's population. Yes, the more reason to detox, but a whole lot easier to find excuses not to detox as well. I tell my clients that if you cannot live without a substance for five weeks then you have a strong addiction and should seek help. The detox program will be an excellent aid in helping you to cleanse your body and reduce any cravings during your treatments.

If you are under a physician's care and are taking medications, continue to take them, but have the dose monitored by your doctor during the course of your detoxification program. You may find that as your blood pressure and cholesterol levels go down, you will need to reduce the medications treating these issues as well. This is something only your doctor can advise you about and not for you to determine by yourself.

Detox Alert

Reducing your intake of medications should only be done under the guidance of a medical doctor. Have your doctor monitor your blood levels during your detox program and adjust medications where necessary.

For the rest of you, giving up your pleasures may involve some discomfort and plenty of reluctance. You are not alone in your attachment to pleasure foods and drinks. However, keep in mind that after you complete your detox program you are free to have those pleasures again. Hopefully by then you will have changed some old habits and developed some healthier ones along the way.

Sweet Nothings

A hundred years ago sugar was an occasional food eaten in holiday desserts and on special occasions. Over time Americans have gone from eating a trace of sugar per year to 150 pounds per person per year. That is equivalent to a national average of 40 teaspoons of sugar per person per day, and has created a national health disaster. We are seeing adult-onset diabetes in adolescents at alarming rates.

These huge amounts of sweetener wreak havoc with an adult's blood sugar. Now just imagine how overwhelming this can be for the body of a small child. It is no mystery that more and more children are developing the adult form of diabetes. This is most likely due in part to high-fructose corn syrup being used in almost every packaged food on your grocery shelves.

In 1997 alone, Americans consumed 7.3 billion pounds of candy and spent an estimated $23.1 billion dollars on candy and gum. As a nation addicted to refined sugar, the cost is reflected in obesity, diabetes, dental problems, and depletion of vital nutrients from the body. Refined sugar is an empty food, lacking fiber, minerals, proteins, fat, and living enzymes. All it contains is calories—and plenty of them.

Regular consumption of sugar lowers your immunity and robs your bones of minerals. This creates conditions that are not worth a lifetime of suffering despite the pleasure of eating sweets:

Healthy Tidbits _____

Your pancreas is designed to handle, in a lifetime, the amount of sugar that most Americans consume in a single month!

- ◆ Irritable bowel syndrome
- ◆ Gallstones and kidney stones
- ◆ Heart disease
- ◆ Cancer
- ◆ Hypoglycemia
- ◆ Insulin resistance
- ◆ Tooth decay

- ◆ Diabetes
- ◆ Skin rashes
- ◆ Obesity
- ◆ Arthritis
- ◆ Aging skin
- ◆ Candida albicans

With a list like that, I think you begin to get the idea that this concentrated food is more deadly than delicious. In fact, because everything of value is removed during the refining process except the high-calorie carbohydrates, and given sugar's extreme concentration, it's considered by many health professionals to be a poison and an addictive drug.

Pure Insights _____

... white refined sugar is not a food. It is a pure chemical extracted from plant sources, purer in fact than cocaine, which it resembles in many ways. Its true name is sucrose and its chemical formula is $C_{12}H_{22}O_{11}$. It has 12 carbon atoms, 22 hydrogen atoms, 11 oxygen atoms, and absolutely nothing else to offer.

—Dr. David Reuben, *Everything You Always Wanted to Know About Nutrition*

Artificial sweeteners are no better and will be eliminated during your detox and hopefully for the rest of your life (see Chapter 2 for more on artificial sweeteners).

I know you love that sweet taste and during your detox there are some high-quality sweeteners you will be allowed to have. This will give you time to transition off the refined sugars gradually without going through a serious sweet tooth withdrawal.

The Caffeine Buzz

Unbeknownst to you, perhaps, the chemical name for caffeine is trimethylxanthine. When isolated in pure form, caffeine is a bitter-tasting white crystalline powder. It is also consumed by 90 percent of the world's population in some form. It is highly addictive, and because of the large amounts consumed to keep up with our fast-paced world, it is considered a modern-day drug.

Caffeine functions in the body using the same mechanisms that amphetamines, cocaine, and heroin use to stimulate the brain. Although milder in its effects, caffeine still manipulates the same neurotransmitters in the brain that give these drugs their addictive qualities.

For years caffeine has been used medicinally as a cardiac stimulant and also as a mild diuretic, because it increases urine production. In our fast-paced, stress-filled lives we use caffeine as an energy boost to create a feeling of heightened alertness. For most of you, a cup of joe provides the jolt you need to function in the morning.

It's an eye-opener to discover just how much caffeine chocolate, herbal sports drinks, and soda all contain. Take a look for yourself:

- 6 oz. of drip-brewed coffee: 100 mg
- 14–20 ounces of coffee: 300 mg
- 6 oz. of black tea: 70 mg
- 7 oz. of green tea: 70 mg
- 12 oz. of Coke, Pepsi, Mountain Dew: 50 mg
- 12 oz. of Jolt: 70 mg
- 12 oz. of Red Bull: 80 mg
- 1 oz. of milk chocolate: 6 mg
- 1 tablet of Anacin: 32 mg

- 1 tablet of No-Doze: 100 mg
- 1 tablet of Vivarin or Dexatrim: 200 mg

An American adult or child on the Standard American Diet can easily consume 300 milligrams of caffeine in a day! How so? Consider for breakfast most people have coffee or tea, perhaps with a chocolate-filled croissant. A common lunch is a sandwich or burger with a cola; a snack might be a handful of M&Ms or chocolate bar and another cup of coffee or cola; and along with your dinner you might have a cola drink. This adds up to a whole lot of stimulants in your bloodstream. No wonder you can't sleep at night! But don't despair. There are still plenty of beverages you can drink, as you'll discover in Chapter 5.

> **Pure Insights**
>
> The problem with caffeine is that the effects can vary, so it is difficult to say what is a safe level. High levels of caffeine can be dangerous for people with high blood pressure or anxiety disorders. Not much is known about taurine and glucuronolactone, but high levels of them could affect the body.
>
> —Dietician Lyndel Costain, speaking about the ingredients in Red Bull, an energy drink

One for the Road

While doing any part of the detox program, you will have to give up drinking alcohol. That glass of wine or two for dinner, the cold beers after work, a dry martini to start the weekend … alcohol is a tough habit to break and an even harder addiction to give up. Considered a poison for the body in some forms, alcohol nonetheless in moderation is beneficial for the heart and arteries. It can all get very confusing, especially after a few drinks.

Alcohol is a high-sugar food and not only feeds yeast, but causes swelling in the joints. Consuming too much of this sugar turns it immediately to fat. Bummer. Drinking alcohol can also dehydrate the body and age the skin. If someone is having more than two alcoholic beverages a day and acting depressed, paranoid, or irritable, the alcohol may be the reason.

> **Healthy Tidbits**
>
> Use your food journal to record what you eat, drink, and the amounts that you consume. At the end of the week you can total up the number of alcohol drinks and grams of caffeine you have had. This will give you an idea as to just how much you are ingesting on a daily basis.

In excess, alcohol is toxic to the liver and can lead to cirrhosis or liver cancer. If you drink alcohol on a regular basis, take a day or two in between drinking to let your liver process the alcohol. The five-week detox program allows for a slow transition off of alcohol to avoid any detox side effects. The good news is that you will be giving all your organs a respite by allowing them time to regenerate and repair.

Smokin' Like a Chimney

The first thing I tell people who refuse to quit smoking is that they are causing a great deal of harm to their body. If they still refuse to quit, the second thing I tell them is to switch to an organic, additive-free light cigarette. It's a first step in lessening the more than 4,000 chemicals in tobacco smoke. Then smoke fewer cigarettes each day, switch to the nicotine patch, and stop smoking altogether. Doing your detox program at the same time creates the perfect conditions for you to quit smoking. Eating a high-quality, high-fiber diet will help your blood to cleanse and ease up on your withdrawal symptoms. Plan to quit smoking when you begin the five-week detox program and let the process unfold one day at a time.

What's Left to Eat?

Your brain is probably working overtime trying to work out whether you can give up all the foods I outlined in this chapter. Having worked with hundreds of people with the same concerns, I can assure you that it is not as difficult as you may think. All the information is provided for you in easy step-by-step progressions.

Today's supermarkets stock many of the organic whole foods you will need. Health-food stores have become natural food supermarkets with one-stop shopping to make it all simple and easy. An interesting fact is that most people rotate only 10 recipes during the course of a given week. Just 10! During detox you will have a chance to break out of your diet rut and explore some new foods and tastes. You will eat plenty of food and experience more variety. All this will cost you is the benefit of feeling great and looking fantastic!

The Least You Need to Know

◆ The Standard American Diet is low in fiber and nutrients, which can weaken your immune system.

◆ Pasteurized dairy products weaken your digestive system.

◆ The main staple in the American diet is white, refined wheat flour, which can cause constipation and intestinal problems.

◆ Refined sugar is an empty food lacking fiber, minerals, proteins, fat, and living enzymes; of all the foods consumed today, sugar is considered the most harmful.

◆ Caffeine, alcohol, and nicotine are addictive drugs and should be transitioned off of slowly to avoid detox side effects.

Chapter 4

Meet Your Organs of Detoxification

In This Chapter

◆ The many tasks your liver performs

◆ Your bloated intestines

◆ How your lungs breathe

◆ Kidneys as vital filters

This is one of the most important chapters in the book because it is all about how you work on the inside. Your physical body operates off a natural intelligence that is astounding in its scope and magnitude. If you ignore its presence and feed it trash, it will work accordingly. However, if you feed your body properly, keep it clean with periodic detoxing, and get regular exercise, your body will last you a good long lifetime.

In this chapter, you are going to meet the tireless workers that keep you functioning day after day. The organs of elimination covered in this chapter include the liver, colon, lungs, and kidneys. Your largest organ of elimination, the skin, is covered in Chapter 20. Now let's get to know them better.

Your Overworked Liver

The liver is your largest solid organ of elimination. It is located on the right side of your body just under the rib cage, between the fifth and sixth ribs. For some reason it has been assigned over 400 tasks on a daily basis. Here are just a few:

- Removes bacteria, fungi, viruses, and parasites from bloodstream
- Metabolizes drugs, chemicals, pesticides, and hormones
- Manufactures 13,000 different enzymes
- Produces cholesterol
- Eliminates excess estrogen
- Regulates blood sugar
- Manufactures bile
- Breaks down old red blood cells

To do all of this the liver requires two sources of blood supply: one from the hepatic artery and one from the portal vein. Blood from the gastrointestinal tract and spleen is then transported through the portal vein and into the liver.

The Liver and Cholesterol

Cholesterol is necessary for the proper function of your internal systems. It is used by the body to build cell membranes and for making certain essential hormones. Triglycerides, on the other hand, are chains of fatty acids that provide energy for your cells to function. It is the liver's job to see that all body tissues receive the right amount of cholesterol and triglycerides to function properly. Your liver produces cholesterol and triglycerides naturally, but you also get them from dietary sources such as animal products and saturated fat. In the digestive process these lipids are taken in through your intestines and delivered to the liver via the bloodstream, where they are processed and re-released as lipoproteins.

There are two forms of lipoproteins:

- *Low-density lipoproteins, known as "bad" LDL.* When levels of these are too high, they tend to stick to the lining of blood vessels, leading to hardening of the arteries. This creates conditions for heart disease and stroke.

◆ *High-density lipoproteins, known as "good" HDL.* Increased levels of HDL act as blood-cell cleaners, scouring the walls and cleaning out excess LDL cholesterol to be returned to the liver for further processing.

A diet high in saturated fat from animal sources can lead to excess levels of "bad" LDL and put you at risk for heart disease. The oils you will be using during the five-week detox program are from plant sources that will supply "good" HDL to strengthen your heart and support your liver function.

Your Liver Knows Detox

Your liver takes care of 75 percent of the body's detoxification, with the additional 25 percent taking place in the intestinal mucosa wall. Detoxification enzymes are present in the tips of the microvilli, the hairlike extensions of the gut wall that absorb nutrients and break them down before absorption.

Intestinal microfloras are the "good guys" in your bowels. A balanced intestinal ecology includes plenty of these probiotics. They produce compounds that promote or inhibit detoxification. Good bacteria encourage detox pathways, while bad bacteria, such as yeast overgrowth, inhibit them.

The liver is a master cleanser. Only your liver can purify the bloodstream, removing toxins, chemicals, fats, and microorganisms. It is your waste treatment plant for removing poisons from your body.

Detox Alert

As their livers detoxify, people are known to become a bit short-tempered and irritable. Try having a cup of milk thistle tea, or put a dropper full of milk thistle tincture into 4 ounces of water and sip slowly. You can purchase milk thistle at most natural foods markets or vitamin stores.

A Dysfunctional Liver

When your liver is healthy, it is a smooth-operating filter. Within your liver there are rows of cells separated by spaces through which the blood flows. These spaces capture the toxins, chemicals, drugs, dead cells, and general debris, just as any filter would work. Your liver also takes on ridding the blood of the underlying microorganisms: bacteria, viruses, fungi, and parasites.

The majority of these chemicals are fat soluble, and it is the liver's job to convert them to water-soluble chemicals. They can then be easily excreted from your body in the form of urine and bile. In order for the liver to do this, it needs certain nutrients to keep it in functioning form. Antioxidants such as vitamins C and E and natural carotenoids in the form of strawberries, red peppers, cold-pressed oils, organic eggs, molasses, leafy green vegetables, nuts, and seeds provide the antioxidants that reduce free radicals and protect the liver cells. It's best to buy organic produce whenever possible to avoid taking in any toxic chemicals from pesticides and herbicides.

Then there are the really harmful chemicals that need to be dealt with in another way. This is handled in the conjugation pathway, a part of the liver where the cells produce substances such as cysteine, glycine, glutamine, choline inositol, and/or sulphur molecules, and adds them to toxins and drugs to render them water soluble. They can then be excreted from the body in the form of urine or bile.

Healthy Tidbits

Scientists have been astounded to find that there are more worlds within worlds in our bodies than are in all the galaxies of the universe. There are millions of functions happening in your body every second of the day. Who is breathing, digesting the food, processing fat, controlling sugar, and feeding blood to the heart while your mind wanders off in daydreams?

To support your liver's valiant efforts you will need a diet that includes foods high in sulphur compounds (garlic, onions, leeks, shallots); cruciferous vegetables (broccoli, cabbage, brussels sprouts, cauliflower); and organic eggs loaded with omega-3 fatty acids. For people with sulpha/sulfa drug allergies, the sulphur compounds in food are a different molecule and you need not worry.

Problems occur when the liver becomes overloaded with debris and cannot turn fat-soluble toxins to water soluble. The pesticides, herbicides, dioxin, and PCBs that are not excreted are then stored in the fatty tissues of your body, such as your brain and endocrine (hormonal) glands and breasts. Many of these carcinogenic chemicals stay there for years, causing problems with brain dysfunction, infertility, menstrual problems, and breast and other cancers.

You can now see why it is so important to keep your liver clean and healthy. Like any filter, your liver needs to be cleansed on a daily basis, and eating a whole-foods diet high in fiber and nutrients is the key here. You can also help it along with the detox program outlined in Part 3 and the liver tonics and herbs, which I describe in Chapter 17.

> ## Pure Insights
>
> Fatty liver occurs when fat accumulation is more than 5 percent of the liver weight. Fatty liver is most commonly caused by incorrect diet, obesity, alcoholism, and diabetes. Other causes can include malnutrition (especially protein deficiency), congenital metabolic disorders, excessive use or toxicity of orthodox medications (such as corticosteroids, valproic acid, tetracycline, salicylates, or synthetic oestrogens), or systemic illnesses with fever.
>
> —Simone Abaron, naturopath

Liver and Weight Loss

Your liver is the major fat-burning organ that attempts to regulate fat metabolism as you scarf down a Big Mac and fries. Your metabolism turns your food energy into cellular energy and the speed in which this happens is called your metabolic rate. If your liver is healthy, your metabolism works quickly, utilizing your intake of food for energy, and your weight remains stable. However, with a sluggish and weak liver, your metabolic rate is lowered, causing food calories to be stored as fat rather than used for energy. Overeating sugar and high-fat or refined foods is a major cause of this problem.

Your Swollen Colon

Food enters through your mouth and hopefully exits out your anus along one long, hollow tube. What happens in between makes the difference in the quality of your health. Digestion begins in your mouth with chewing your food. Breaking down the fibers in food, while enzymes are released in the saliva, is crucial for the next stage. Once swallowed, the food passes into the stomach, where it is mixed with hydrochloric acid and further broken down. It then passes into your small intestine, which at 20 feet long, has three sections working different jobs to absorb nutrients.

The duodenum mixes the food from the stomach with bile from the liver and gallbladder. This helps to break down fats. The pancreas contributes digestive enzymes and the food moves along to the jejunum. Your life, literally, depends on this phase of digestion. Here the molecular-size nutrients are extracted by the lumen of the small intestine and absorbed by the lining cells and transferred to blood and lymph capillaries for eventual delivery to the liver for processing.

If your small intestine is unable to extract the vitamins, minerals, and protein from the food, your tissues and cells will starve, leading to fatigue, degeneration, and eventually disease.

Meanwhile, any undigested material is moved through the ileum and into the large intestine. Water and minerals are extracted and the leftover waste is pushed through the anal canal and eliminated through the anus. Simple, brilliant, and effective—when it is all working properly.

When Your Belly Hurts

Gas, bloating, and intestinal distress can be painful and uncomfortable for you and anyone unfortunate enough to be standing nearby. The three major causes of this distress are …

- ◆ Poor diet.

- ◆ Overgrowth of unfriendly microorganisms.

- ◆ Stress.

If the liver and pancreas are not functioning properly, this can lead to poor digestion of food and improper absorption of nutrients, not to mention the undigested condition of the food once it reaches the large intestine. If your large intestine could talk, it might say to those other organs: "Great. Hey thanks, guys, more work for me to do. What am I supposed to do with these huge chunks of meat? I am not designed to handle this."

We need to take a moment and talk about all that mucus in your system. Mucus is that slippery, runny substance that exits your body during a good head cold. It does, however, play an important role by protecting delicate membrane tissue and trapping toxins to eliminate them from your body. Too much mucus can coat the intestinal walls in such a way that toxins and fecal debris accumulate, creating the ideal environment for trouble down below. Mucus-forming foods include the following:

- ◆ Dairy products

- ◆ Animal protein

- ◆ White flour

- ◆ Processed foods

- ◆ Chocolate

- ◆ Coffee

- ◆ Alcohol

This thick accumulation of mucus, combined with poor digestive ability and a lack of friendly microorganisms, can create an overgrowth of yeast and parasites in your gut.

Now you have a real mess, and that's speaking politely. Inflammation, sores, cysts, ulcers, polyps, and constipation and/or diarrhea are a few of the results. The good news is that once you are no longer eating the foods that cause your problems and you are cleansing your intestines according to the detox program in Part 3, you will be on your way to recovering your health and your sanity as well.

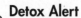

Detox Alert _____

Just because you find them in the dairy section of your grocery store, don't mistake eggs for a dairy product. They are an animal protein. Dairy foods are made from the milk of the mammary gland of female mammals.

The Underlying Organisms

Living in your gut is an odd assortment of organisms. Yeast, parasites, friendly and unfriendly bacteria, and viruses are the central characters. In this environment the friendly beneficial microflora keep everyone else under control. They propagate good flora, keeping your intestinal ecology healthy and balanced. Imbalance occurs from taking antibiotics, birth-control pills, chlorinated water, or cortisone drugs, and eating a nutritiously empty SAD diet (see Chapter 3). These chemicals and drugs kill off the "good guys," leaving the yeast, parasites, viruses, and bad bacteria plenty of space to multiply and take over.

Candida Albicans

Many people suffer from an overgrowth of yeast and don't know that this is the underlying cause of their symptoms. Known as *Candida albicans*, it is a common health problem for women, men, and children. It weakens your immune system, creating vitamin/mineral deficiencies and an acid blood condition. There are a broad range of Candida-inspired symptoms; some of the most common are:

def•i•ni•tion _____

Candida albicans is an overgrowth of yeast organisms in the GI tract. They feed on sugar, refined carbohydrates, fermented foods, alcohol, and dairy products.

- Foggy brain, poor memory, spacey feeling

- Abdominal bloating, gas, pain

- Fatigue

- Insomnia

- Diarrhea and/or constipation

- Vaginal or penile itching

- Vaginal discharge

- Endometriosis

- Inability to lose weight

- Joint pains

To bring the yeast organisms under control and reestablish the beneficial microflora requires following a strict antifungal diet and taking probiotics rich in beneficial microflora. Herbal supplements that help starve yeast and eliminate it from the body are garlic, caprylic acid, Pau D'Arco, oregano oil, and olive leaf. Colloidal silver is also used to control yeast as it is antifungal.

If you feel you have this condition, your detox program will help to address it on a surface level, but you will need to go deeper in the healing process with the guidance of a certified nutritionist or medical doctor.

Parasites

You might not like the idea of bugs and worms moving around in your bowels, but those raw salads you buy from the local deli, a trip to Cancun or other exotic locales, and unfiltered well water can all contribute to invading foreigners taking a swim down your digestive track. The problem is they stick around in that nice warm environment where they're provided with plenty of food to eat. Why go anywhere else? They lay their eggs, socialize, and begin to wreak havoc with your digestive system.

Many of the symptoms for parasite infestation mimic the Candida symptoms: bloating, constipation, diarrhea, gas, and fatigue. When specific treatment for irritable bowel syndrome (IBS) doesn't work, parasites might be the problem. You can have your doctor analyze a stool sample, but this doesn't always reveal the little critters. Better testing is available, but you may need to find a holistic practitioner with some experience in dealing with parasites.

> **Pure Insights** _____
>
> It is now my belief that IBS is just the beginning of the story, not the conclusion. Because of my own experience with GI distress, I now test for parasites in every woman who comes into the clinic with a diagnosis or symptoms of IBS. You may be surprised to learn that 40 percent of these women prove to have intestinal parasites—even though many have never left the United States.
>
> —Dr. Marcelle Pick, OB/GYN, nurse practitioner, and registered nurse

Health-food stores are awash with parasite-cleansing kits. These kits include packets of herbal supplements that normally cover a 10-day regimen. It is suggested that you then take a 7- to 10-day break and repeat the parasite-cleansing process. This ensures that you kill off and eliminate any eggs that may have stayed behind from the first round of supplements. You may be sensitive to the laxatives used in some of these kits, so before buying check with a certified health practitioner to ensure you are taking a safe and effective product.

During the detox program, many of your symptoms will ease up and some parasites may be eliminated—but not all. You will need to follow a parasite detox protocol, which I outline in Chapter 17. If you add this to your five-week detox program, you can kill two parasites with one stone, or so the saying goes.

Detox Your Way to Health

The organisms living in your large intestine are kept under control by the friendly microflora, acidophilus and bifidus. These probiotics help to stabilize and balance the ecology in your bowels. In 1928, bacteriologist Alexander Fleming accidentally discovered the first antibiotic, and our bowels were changed forever. Antibiotics are wonder drugs that destroy deadly bacteria and save lives, but at the same time they wipe out friendly probiotics, leaving the bowels susceptible to an overgrowth of yeast, parasites, and viruses. The proverbial catch-22—damned if you do, damned if you don't.

> **Pure Insights** _____
>
> I estimate that more than half the adults in the United States are digesting and absorbing less than half of what they eat.
>
> —Robert O. Young, Ph.D., *The pH Miracle*

Replanting your intestines with probiotics during and after taking antibiotics is necessary to rebalance and heal your bowels. (You should take probiotics two hours after taking the antibiotic, so as not to interfere with its efficacy.) It's also necessary to eliminate refined foods, sugar, alcohol, moldy or pickled foods, dried fruits, and yeast extracts from your diet. In addition, you should detoxify your intestines and replant acidophilus and bifidus using raw fermented sauerkrauts and raw, unfiltered apple cider vinegar. It will take some time and effort, but you can return your organs to health in this manner.

Your Laboring Lungs

In Eastern medicine the lungs and large intestine have a strong connection. Overabundance of mucus rises up from the intestines and into the lungs, eventually moving into the sinuses blocking the passageway or making a run for it out your nostrils. Some mucus is necessary to trap toxins in the lungs to be expelled by coughing. Your lungs eliminate carbon dioxide when breathing while also expelling any poisonous gases taken in through the breathing process.

Counting Your Breath

There are many breathing exercises you can do to cleanse your lungs. They are worth practicing because they increase your oxygen levels, help to calm the nervous system, and stabilize your mind. They also increase your lung capacity, allowing for more *prana* (life force) to feed the body's vital energy. The following breathing exercise will help you increase your oxygen intake while cleansing your lungs.

def•i•ni•tion

Prana is a Sanskrit word which translates as both breath and life. It is the vital energy force that pervades our physical, mental, and spiritual bodies, keeping us alive and vibrant.

Try sitting quietly in a chair, your feet on the floor, with your hands relaxed on your thighs. Close your eyes and focus on your breath. Step back in your mind and become the observer. Your thoughts will want to intrude, but stay focused and notice the length of your inhale, then notice the length of your exhale. After a few moments of this, slowly begin counting (in your mind) to four as you inhale and to six as you exhale. Time your breath to begin on the first count and end on the last count. Do six sets of inhale/exhale then relax and breathe normally, without forcing or imposing your will upon your breathing.

Over time you can increase the length of the inhale to a six count and your exhale to an eight count. As your lung capacity expands, increase to an 8-count inhale, 10-count exhale. Advance according to your body's ability to respond comfortably. Never force or push your body to do anything it is unable or unwilling to do. Practice this simple but effective exercise for a few minutes every day.

Alternate Nostril Breathing

Alternate nostril breathing has been practiced for centuries by yogis worldwide. Practiced daily, it will balance the right and left hemispheres of your brain, lower high blood pressure, and balance the brain's serotonin levels, the chemical that regulates your moods.

Using your right hand, touch the tips of your index and middle finger to a point just below the right thumb. Keep your thumb, ring, and little finger extended. Inhale through both nostrils then close your right nostril gently with your right thumb and exhale through your left nostril. Inhale through your left nostril and press it closed with your ring/little finger, lift your thumb and exhale through your right nostril. Inhale through your right, close with your thumb, lift your ring/little fingers and exhale through the left. Go back and forth like this for 6 sets (12 repetitions), then sit and breathe normally for 3 breaths. For your second cycle repeat the sequence but begin by closing the left nostril first.

Begin doing the practice once per day and see if you can increase it to two or three times a day for maximum benefit. You can do it in the quiet of your home, or during a break at work. You will notice that one nostril is always more closed than the other. This is normal because they alternate back and forth every 90 minutes. You can time your breaths by counting in the same way as explained previously.

Kidneys, Your Water Babies

Your kidneys are two ear-shaped organs located just below your rib cage, on either side of your spine. Small but efficient, they are able to process 20 percent of the blood pumped by your heart. They filter waste from your blood (ammonia, drugs, chemicals, urea, toxins), and excrete them through your urine. Your kidneys regulate blood pressure, maintain calcium levels, balance water volume, and keep the acid concentration of your blood constant.

Healthy Tidbits _____

You can prevent diabetes-related kidney problems by keeping your blood glucose close to normal and keeping your blood pressure below 130/80.

Too much sugar in your blood can lead to kidney complications from diabetes. Maintaining a high blood glucose (blood sugar) level has a damaging effect on all your organs, but especially your heart, blood vessels, eyes, and kidneys. Controlling your blood pressure will slow down or prevent damage to these parts of your body.

It is recommended that the best thing you can do to prevent diabetes is to eat a healthy whole-foods diet, just like you will be following on your detox program. Also consider doing a periodic kidney flush, as outlined in Chapter 18.

The Least You Need to Know

◆ The liver is your largest solid organ of elimination and takes care of 75 percent of the all detoxification.

◆ Your life depends on your small intestine's ability to absorb vitamins, minerals, and protein from the food you've eaten.

◆ Following a daily practice of alternate nostril breathing helps to regulate your blood pressure.

◆ Your kidneys filter waste from the blood, regulate blood pressure, maintain calcium levels, and balance water volume, all while keeping the acid concentration of your blood constant.

Part 2

Preparing to Detoxify

Previous chapters showed you that with all the pollutants in our air, food, and water, staying healthy is a challenge everyone on this planet needs to address. For health purposes, one solution is to periodically detoxify your body. This is not only necessary but essential for keeping your organs running clean and doing their jobs properly.

Now let's get you ready for the next step of your detoxing journey. All the essentials you will need—from supplements to cleansing products, food, teas, and encouragement—can be found in these next four chapters. Be sure to read them over carefully before moving on to Part 3. Knowledge is power!

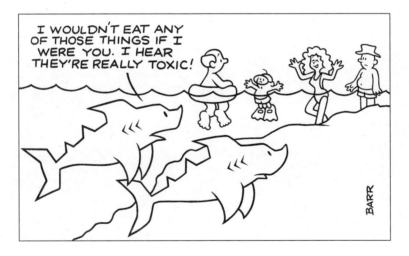

Chapter 5

Getting Off to a Great Start

In This Chapter

- ◆ Choosing a detox program
- ◆ Planning your meals, at home and when eating out
- ◆ Giving your pantry an overhaul
- ◆ The importance of drinking plenty of pure water
- ◆ Other healthy drink options
- ◆ Eating only the best

Choosing the right program for you can be determined by your previous detoxification experience, time constraints, health situation, and willingness to transition to a healthier lifestyle. There are ways to find food outside your kitchen to eat, foods you can take along to work, and even meals that travel long distances with you.

This chapter contains all the information you will need to organize, plan meals, arrange your kitchen, and buy your food. So what are you waiting for? Let's get going!

Choosing Your Detox Program

In Part 4, you will find detox programs ranging from seasonal to a three-day weekend, with the option to do a one-day fast. I suggest, however, that you begin with the five-week detox program, especially if you …

♦ Are just beginning to change your diet.

♦ Want a detox that goes deeper than most others.

♦ Are healing from illness and need to rebuild your depleted system.

The beauty of taking five weeks to detoxify is to allow time for your organs to relax and let go, for your blood to cleanse and your cells to repair themselves. Five weeks is plenty of time to change old habits and establish new ones. Given the advantage of time you can learn about new foods, find your way around the modern natural foods market, and come to terms with any physical changes you are experiencing.

Chapter 9 introduces you to week one of the detox program. Instead of throwing you into food deprivation, it guides you to eliminate one food every few days, with lists of the great foods you can replace them with.

Once the initial awkwardness of starting something new has passed, you will find the first two weeks are pretty easy. Many of your symptoms will have eased, your clothes may feel looser, and your sugar cravings will be gone. That's only the beginning!

Once you've completed the five weeks you will have a better understanding of how to move from trashing your body with low-quality food to eating nutrient-dense foods that only make you look and feel great.

Planning Your Meals

One of the realities of taking responsibility for your health is making sure that the right foods are available at the right times of day. This means you will need to give some thought to planning your meals. Fast food came into being because you didn't have time to think about shopping, planning, and preparing three meals a day. But with fast food comes degeneration and disease. Weigh that against taking a few minutes to plan ahead, and I think you will agree it is worth taking the time.

I suggest you memorize what your daily menu should include in terms of main food groups, protein, carbohydrates, and fats. This balance will ensure you receive all the daily essential nutrients you will need. Make a copy of the following list and use it as a reference when in doubt.

This is for the average adult doing light to moderate exercise:

> 5 servings of vegetables: nonstarchy green, red, orange
>
> 3 to 4 servings of whole grains, cereals, starchy vegetables, and wheat-free flour products
>
> 2 to 3 servings of legumes, beans, peas, lentils, tofu, tempeh, miso
>
> 2 servings of fresh or cooked fruit
>
> 1 to 2 small servings of nuts and seeds
>
> 1 to 2 servings of animal products: eggs, fish, fowl, meat (no pork)
>
> 1 to 2 tablespoons of flax seed oil
>
> 1 to 2 capsules of high-quality cod liver oil
>
> 6 to 8 glasses of pure, clean water

Healthy Tidbits

The best way to determine serving size is protein the size of your palm (4–5 ounces), vegetables the size of your hand, and oil the size of your thumb. (See Chapter 6 for more about protein.)

Chapters 9 through 13 contain lists of foods for detox-appropriate recipes you will find in Appendix B. You may find that you are eating more than you normally do, yet your cravings will lessen and you will lose weight.

Dining Out

When dining out, choose a restaurant that serves plenty of vegetables and is willing to prepare food according to your request. When ordering, ask the waitress for some grilled salmon and vegetables or a grilled vegetable platter. I have had some of my best meals when ordering off the menu in this way.

Detox Alert

When dining out, avoid fried foods, sweetened coffee drinks, cookies, bread and pastries made with refined wheat flour, raw fish, artificial sweeteners, and especially nonorganic wine. Grapes are one of the most highly pesticide-sprayed foods, which can concentrate in the wine. There are some excellent organic wines available for your drinking pleasure that are well worth trying.

If you are a regular to the restaurant, bring along a package of wheat-free pasta and ask the chef to prepare it with olive oil and garlic. Pack a small container of home-made salad dressing and carry it in your purse. Bring a few dates and walnuts to have for dessert and order a cup of hot water and lemon to sip.

Some restaurants are easier than others to find a detox-friendly meal. Consider these menu ideas when dining out:

- Japanese: Brown rice and vegetables, stir-fried vegetables with fish, rolls with cooked fish, miso soup, soba noodles in miso broth. Avoid soy sauce as it contains wheat and has a high sodium content.

- Diner: Vegetable omelet, grilled chicken or fish over salad greens, and stir-fried or steamed vegetables.

- Chinese: Vegetable bean curd soup, steamed vegetables with chicken or fish. Avoid soy or white sauce. Ask for your dish steamed or lightly sautéed with garlic and ginger.

- Grill: Fish and vegetables, grilled chicken or shrimp over salad with oil and vinegar, grilled vegetable platter.

Unless it states on the menu that the ingredients are organically raised, you can bet they've been sprayed and contain additives. Work it out the best way you can, because you can't always control what there is to eat outside your own kitchen. Perhaps one day all our food will be clean and nutritious. Until then we make compromises when necessary.

Your Lunch Box

Exactly where are you at lunchtime? If you're at the office and eat out regularly, you can choose to pack a healthy lunch, or consider the previous suggestions. Cafeteria food probably won't accommodate your detox, unless the chef is kind enough to prepare it especially for you. I know people who hand their company chef their detox recipes and they appear on the next day's menu. If enough people in your office are following the detox program, the chef may make the effort. There's no harm in asking.

If possible, install a small refrigerator in the office lounge. This will make it more convenient to bring your lunch. You can also set up a blender to make healthy smoothies for a quick snack or light meal. This way you can have the best food available, and it will save you money over time. If you spend a lot of time at the office, make it feel like home. Keep food in the fridge and an electric tea pot for heating water. If you don't take care of your own needs, I can assure you, no one else will.

Detox Alert

Avoid using a microwave oven. Microwave radiation interacts with the molecules in food. All this agitation creates molecular "friction," which heats up the food. This unusual type of heating also causes substantial damage to the surrounding molecules, often tearing them apart or forcefully deforming them. This friction type of energy can be transmitted from your food to your body, adding another kind of agitation to your overtaxed nervous system.

Traveling Meals

During a recent trip, I was high in the air and the flight attendants were pushing the food cart down the center aisle. I reached under the seat in front of me and lifted my food container onto my tray. I then proceeded to set out four containers of my home-cooked meal. The couple across the aisle kept glancing from my food to their airplane food. Finally the husband leaned across the aisle and said, "That's a great idea. I wish we had done it ourselves." I told him it was easy to do, gave him a few tips, and we both went back to chewing.

I always bring along food when traveling, whether taking a cooler loaded with essentials in my car or my trusty Nissan jar. The Nissan jar is a stainless-steel cylinder with four small containers, each one with a different dish, such as salad, grains, protein, and something sweet. On the return trip I refill my containers so I will have the kind of meal I need, no matter where I find myself. In my carry-on, I stash my sweeteners, xylitol and stevia, along with my morning tea, some toasted almonds, and raisins. You never know what can happen when traveling, so being prepared is not just for Boy or Girl Scouts.

The old lunch box has morphed into a lightweight cold pack with several food compartments. These are great to take along when traveling. Some other ideas for travel food:

- A thermos with hot soup, some raw veggies, and a bag of spelt crackers makes a quick meal.

- Cooked brown rice combined with diced carrots, red onion, toasted sunflower seeds, black beans, and chopped spinach can be tossed with an olive oil vinaigrette and served out of lidded glass containers. Fantastic!

- A spelt tortilla spread with hummus, salad greens, and the grain quinoa makes a great wrap.

- Pancakes you make one day can double as snack cakes the next.

All you need to let your taste buds run free is the list of ingredients and a bit of imagination. You can travel and stay on your detox program with just a little bit of extra effort. Believe me, it's worth it.

Family Holidays

Give up all hope, all ye who enter here. Family holidays are not the time to be doing a detox program. Planning family meals around your special considerations will only make life difficult for everyone. If you show up and tell them you are eating organic vegetables and protein rather than barbecue pork ribs, lasagna, red-velvet chocolate cake, or multiple kegs of beer, you are asking to be the life of the party, at your expense.

I strongly suggest you detox before you party with your family. This way you show up looking fabulous, skin glowing, swelling down in the ankles, and fitting into your old jeans. What can I tell you, life is made up of moments like this!

Purging Your Pantry

If it's not on the detox food list, then you don't want it around. Foods for other family members can be placed in a cabinet just for them. Take over a space in the kitchen to store the foods you will be eating during the five-week program. Little by little you can substitute some of your children's high-sugar cereals with healthier brands.

I know for a fact that if a food you cannot resist eating is anywhere in the house, you will eat it. Give those foods away to neighbors, friends, or the local food bank. Purchase a version of the foods you love that are made with organic ingredients, ones that contribute vital nutrients for your body to utilize. Entertainment food such as chips, candy, baked desserts, and "healthy" junk food only provides extra calories and fats that you don't need. Instead, try the meal and snack ideas located in Chapters 9 through 13 and Appendix B.

Getting Plenty of Water

Your body is 75 percent water, a liquid vital for keeping your body running effectively. Believe it or not, a loss of just 15 to 20 percent of your body's water can be fatal! You can survive weeks without food, a few days without water, and only a few minutes without breath. Water is one of the three major components that keep you alive, and it is estimated that 75 percent of people are chronically dehydrated. Not drinking enough water prevents your body from utilizing the food you eat and the supplements you take. Naturally, this leads to malnutrition, degeneration, and illness.

Unfortunately, dehydration is often overlooked when diagnosing the cause of these ailments to which it contributes:

> **Healthy Tidbits**
>
> A study at John Hopkins Medical Institution compared 83 people who ate 8 to 10 servings of fruits and vegetables per day, to 40 others who ate fewer servings. The blood of those eating more vegetables had a higher oxidative capacity.

- ◆ Indigestion
- ◆ Colitis
- ◆ Appendicitis
- ◆ Heartburn
- ◆ Rheumatoid arthritis
- ◆ Back and neck pain
- ◆ Headaches

- ◆ Stress
- ◆ Depression
- ◆ High blood pressure
- ◆ Asthma
- ◆ Fatigue
- ◆ Memory loss
- ◆ Allergies

Pure Insights

I have had clients gain as much as 8 pounds in water weight as they began to drink more water. I coach them not to back off when this happens. Once their water-starved body consistently gets what it needs, the newly gained water weight falls off, usually in a short period of time.

—Dian Freeman, clinical nutritionist

Water helps to flush the body of disease-causing acid waste products, and drinking 8 to 10 glasses of water per day can significantly reduce back and joint pain. Because your brain is 80 percent water, dehydration can lead to fuzzy, cloudy thinking and trigger short-term memory loss. Do not wait until your mouth is dry to drink water. This will only stress your body's system. You need to be drinking pure filtered or spring water at regular intervals throughout the day.

It is recommended that a healthy person drink six to eight glasses of water per day, but this does not take into account your size and body weight. Some nutritionists insist you drink one half of your body weight in ounces each day. To determine this, take your current body weight and divide that amount by two. The total will be the minimum number of ounces that your body requires to sustain optimal health. For example: 150 pounds divided by 2 equals 75 ounces, or approximately nine 8-ounce glasses of water per day. This allows for a more realistic estimate for what you, as an individual, will need.

You can get some of your water intake by drinking herbal teas and soup broths. Soaking and cooking your grains in water also provides an absorbable amount of liquid to your system. Your body absorbs only 4 ounces of water at a time, which goes right into your tissues. Drink this amount every half-hour for maximum benefit.

What Else Can You Drink?

If you are used to drinking soda pop or fruit juice as your primary fluid, then you're probably wondering what else there is to drink. I know, water is fine and you've read all the data about getting enough, but to give up your Dr Pepper—well, that's asking a lot. I suggest you learn about what you are drinking. In this way you will understand why you need to make a switch.

Teenagers are the fastest-growing group in the United States developing osteoporosis. Yes, teenagers. Much of this is due to their large consumption of soda pop. I understand that this is hard to believe when deterioration of the bones is associated more with older women. However, with the amount of pop that teenagers consume on a daily basis, osteoporosis is the inevitable outcome. One look at the ingredients will tell you why:

- Caffeine: inhibits absorption of calcium, causes dehydration

- Carbonated water: decreases blood oxygen by 25 percent for three hours after drinking

- Phosphoric acid: too much leaches calcium from bones

- High-fructose corn syrup: causes dehydration and depletion of minerals, and lowers immune function

Detox Alert

Cola has uses other than for drinking. It can be used to clean toilet bowls, remove rust spots, and clean rusty bolts. It is excellent for cleaning the engines of cars and trucks, and the highway patrol uses it to clean blood off the pavement.

- Aspartame: a dangerous neurotoxin causes multiple physical and mental problems

- Acesulfame k: a toxic poison, causes cancer in test animals

- Sucralose: breaks down to a chemical similar to chlorinated pesticides, 1,6–dichlorofructose.

Talk about a chemical cocktail! To top it off, most of those ingredients are addictive substances. But the question to ask is, how does soda pop leach calcium from your bones?

Your normal blood pH is between 7.2 and 7.4. However, after just one can of either diet or regular soda, you would need 32 glasses of alkalinized water, with a pH of 9, to neutralize what you just drank. Now because you usually don't chase that soda with 32 glasses of alkaline water, your body buffers all that acid by pulling the calcium from your bones—20 milligrams of calcium to be exact, for every can of soda. It's that survival thing again. Your body will try to survive regardless of what you feed it.

Maybe you don't drink soda pop. Instead, you drink orange juice in the morning and cranberry juice to keep your bladder healthy. Good for you. No doubt you are trying to drink more health-promoting beverages; however, there is something else to consider.

Fruit juice has become the latest "it" food and is marketed to young mothers concerned about the health of their small children. It is important to note that soft-drink companies manufacture these juice products. They package the juice in cute little

def•i•ni•tion

Pasteurization is the process of heating liquids to a high temperature in order to destroy any harmful organisms, such as viruses, bacteria, protozoa, molds, and yeasts. The process also destroys beneficial nutrients and enzymes in the liquids. In the case of fruit and vegetable juice, you are left with a high-sugar beverage without the fiber.

colorful boxes and kids drink them all day long, not just for breakfast. Because the juice has been *pasteurized*, anything that was once good and healthy is no longer present.

There are 6 teaspoons of sugar in 8 ounces of fruit juice. This will cause the same rise in insulin levels that you get from refined white sugar. Plus, many of these fruit juices are supplemented with synthetic vitamins to appear more appealing. After drinking four or five containers of juice in a day, the liver and pancreas have been seriously stressed. This distortion of insulin balance may lead to hormone and neurotransmitter shifts, which could increase the risk of ear infections, allergies, and ADHD.

I suggest you purchase a good juicing machine and juice organic fruit and vegetables fresh daily. Fresh juice provides immediate nutrients to your body; the variety of combinations is endless and the taste is much better than the processed brands.

You can also have nondairy milks such as soy, rice, almond, oat, and hazelnut. These milks are delicious and go well on cereal, in coffee, and to make creamy soups. Coming off of coffee during your first two weeks, you should try having an organic soy decaf latte. Many popular coffee bars carry soy or rice milk, providing their customers with healthier choices.

Pure Insights

Nature has provided us with the answers for preventing health problems. I do not recommend pasteurized orange juice or reconstituted juice of any kind. The greatest health benefits are derived from drinking raw, fresh fruit and vegetable juices, straight from nature.

—Mike Adams, *The Seven Laws of Nutrition*

The varieties of organic teas on the market will keep you endlessly entertained experimenting with taste. You can use green tea to help with the caffeine withdrawal from coffee during the first week of your detox program. Then switch to decaffeinated green tea, or try dandelion, burdock, or nettle tea, which will help your liver detoxify gently.

Unsweetened cranberry juice diluted with water and sweetened with the herb stevia is a good substitute for the commercial sugar-sweetened brands. Try some in a wine glass when you want the appearance of having red wine. You can feel comfortable dining with people who won't know the difference.

Coffee and black tea have diuretic properties that can lead to dehydration when consumed in excess. (A diuretic is an herb, plant, or chemical that releases fluids from the body.) They are also considered acid-forming to your blood pH. Disease grows in an acid condition. Drink minimal amounts or not at all. Grain coffee substitutes are very satisfying taste-wise, but without the caffeine kick. They are made from grains, fruit, and some nuts, all ground and roasted. Some can be brewed in a coffee brewer and some come as an instant beverage that can be transformed with boiling water.

The most beneficial detox drink is the juice of half a lemon mixed with 8 ounces of water and sweetened to taste. Freshly squeezed lemon juice is the perfect way to begin your morning and end your night. Lemon juice works by softening the liver so it can release trapped toxins and chemicals. (After drinking fresh lemon juice, rinse your mouth with pure water or brush your teeth. The acidity of lemons can be abrasive to tooth enamel.)

Eat Organically Grown Foods

Many of the toxins and chemicals in your system are coming from the foods you eat and drink. If you are trying to eliminate them from your organs, then it is not a good idea to be putting them back into your body. Eating organically raised fruits, vegetables, grains, beans, nuts, seeds, along with organic, grass-fed beef and poultry is recommended when doing your detox program.

It is important not to be fooled when shopping for healthier, cleaner food. The *organic* food market is growing at a rate of 20 percent a year, a huge shift from 30 years ago when I first began changing my way of eating. Change is happening slowly, but it is happening.

def•i•ni•tion

> **Organic** refers to crops grown without chemical pesticides or chemical fertilizers. Animals are raised without drugging them with hormones or antibiotics. Sewage sludge is not allowed to be spread on farmlands. You cannot feed animals things like blood, slaughterhouse waste, manure, and municipal garbage, and you cannot use untested and hazardous technologies like genetic engineering or food irradiation.

Whole Foods has listed the 11 "best reasons to buy organic" on the sides of its grocery bags:

1. Organic farming meets the needs of the present without compromising the needs of future generations.

2. Growing organically supports a biologically diverse, healthy environment.

3. Organic farming practices help protect our water resources.

4. Organic agriculture increases the land's productivity.

5. Organic production limits toxic and long-lasting chemicals in our environment.

6. Buying organic supports small, independent family farms.

7. Organic farmers are less reliant on nonrenewable fossil fuels.

8. Organic products meet stringent USDA standards.

9. Buying organic is a direct investment in the long-term future of our planet.

10. Organic farmers preserve diversity of plant species.

11. Organic food tastes great.

Eating organic foods is better for your health. Knowing this, the American consumer is responding to the need for higher-quality foods. Unfortunately, agri-business is stepping in to change the rules and control the meaning of the word "organic." What was once pure, whole foods from healthy soil and animals may come to be no better than what has always been offered: depleted soils, cancer-causing fruits and vegetables, abusive animal conditions, and a toxic environment.

The health of our food supply is the most important issue the world has to contend with at this time. Without clean, healthy food we will only see more debilitation in the physical health of human beings. As you experience the benefits of eating an organic, whole foods diet, you will want to know what you can do to help create a cleaner, healthier food supply:

- Seek out local organic farmers and buy from them.

- Join your local community-supported garden.

- Learn how to grow organic food at home.

- Demand that your grocery and health-food stores carry humanely raised meats and poultry.

- Stay current on what is happening in Congress concerning food bills.

- Contact your state's congressmen and let them know how you feel about keeping your food safe.

It is your dollar that does the talking, so spend it wisely. You'll not only get the best, but you will have an impact on the health of our planet as well.

The Least You Need to Know

- The right program should be determined by your previous detoxification experience, time constraints, health situation, and willingness to transition to a healthier lifestyle.

- Take a few minutes out of each day to plan your meals and make a shopping list.

- When dining out, choose a restaurant that serves plenty of vegetables and is willing to prepare food according to your request.

- Drinking 8 to 10 glasses of pure filtered or spring water each day helps to flush the body of acid waste products and can significantly reduce back and joint pain.

- Freshly squeezed lemon juice mixed with water is the perfect way to begin and end your day, while softening the liver enough to release trapped toxins and chemicals.

- Whenever possible, buy organic foods for the best detox results.

What You Will Need to Detox

In This Chapter

- ◆ Support for your detox
- ◆ The importance of protein
- ◆ Taking vitamins and minerals
- ◆ Supercleansing foods to have on hand
- ◆ Replenishing your intestines

As you will learn in Chapter 11, there are ways to detox that require only distilled water and a place to rest. Getting to that point calls for support along the way. You will need knowledge of your protein requirements, necessary vitamins and minerals, supplements, and cleansing foods that will help you go deeper.

In this chapter, you will find the supporting items to complete your detox program. The food and detoxing techniques are laid out for you in Chapters 9 through 13. Here I discuss the essentials you will want to have on hand or have knowledge about before beginning the program.

Time for Yourself

The experience of detoxing your body can be a very personal one. It is a time of physical change and mental reflection. Taking time for yourself during the next few weeks will enhance the effects of your detox. I recommend you avoid people whom you think might try to sabotage your efforts or make jokes about what you are eating. I would even suggest that you only tell those people close to you what you are doing and invite them to join you in doing the five-week detox program. Having someone to share your experience with can be very supportive. And go ahead, eat out with your friends, just don't make a big deal out of the food you order (see Chapter 5 for some ideas on what to order out).

The Right Protein

Proteins are the building blocks of your body. Twenty percent of our weight is made up of protein. Your muscles, hair, nails, skin, and eyes are mostly protein. It is of tremendous importance because it provides support for your cells, and builds and repairs muscles and other body tissues. The right kind of protein for your blood type and lifestyle can vary from person to person. It is important to take into consideration your daily expenditure of energy and the quality of protein you will need to support this expenditure.

Healthy Tidbits _____

According to Dr. Peter D'Adamo, author of *Eat Right 4 Your Type*, your blood type is the key to your body's entire immune system. Years of research have shown him how each blood type responds to a particular food:

- O blood types should eat a higher purine protein (red meats, lamb, buffalo) and lower carbohydrates. No wheat or dairy.
- A blood types can be vegetarians and do well on higher carbohydrates and low fat.
- B blood types have the most varied diet of all four types, but should avoid chicken.
- AB blood types have the benefits and sensitivities of both the A and B types.

The surgeon general has determined that a 120- to 125-pound person needs a minimum of 60 to 65 grams of protein per day. This can consist of eggs, soybeans, tofu, tempeh, whole grains, meat, fish, poultry, beans, nuts, seeds, milk, and cheese (though not while detoxing). Incomplete proteins such as whole grains and beans, when combined in a meal, become a complete protein. Many ethnic diets are based on a rice, cheese, and bean combination to create a complete protein meal.

Protein should make up about 15 to 20 percent of your daily calories. This translates to 4 ounces (the size of a deck of cards) per meal. In our fast-food culture, grabbing a big burger or 16-ounce steak seems normal, but it is too much protein for your body to digest in one sitting. Instead, eat smaller portions spread over four to six meals.

Supplements

As you learned in Chapter 3, the Standard American Diet is so highly processed that only 25 to 75 percent of the original nutrients remain in the food. Under these conditions, vitamin deficiency can occur even while eating a balanced diet. For example, U.S. government surveys show that the average American diet provides only 40 percent of magnesium per day. Adequate amounts of magnesium are vital to your survival. As a matter of fact, magnesium deficiency can be a cause of sudden cardiac death.

Many commercial vitamins touted in magazine and TV ads as the perfect one-a-day supplement are actually well below normal for optimal nutrient content. Plus, the most powerful antioxidants, CoQ10, grape seed extract, and green tea extract, are missing altogether! The calcium and magnesium used in these supplements are usually inorganic, nonchelated forms and fall below the RDA recommended levels. To stop bone loss, at least 500 to 1500 milligrams of calcium citrate per day are necessary.

Another consideration concerns your digestive system's ability to break down those hard, solid pills. One sewage treatment plant manager told how the plant's water filters are constantly clogged with vitamin tablets. What you swallow, if not properly digested, goes right through the digestive tube and out the other end.

Nutrients You Are Lacking

Thirty percent of the calories Americans consume daily are from the top 10 worst foods for you (see Chapter 3). This means that if you are eating foods with few nutrients, you are lacking crucial vitamins and minerals. If the purpose in eating is to provide nutrient sustenance to your body, then "Houston, we have a problem."

Surprisingly, you can be overweight and still be malnourished. Remember, your body's sole purpose is to survive. When you don't feed it the nutrients it needs, it will

Detox Alert

According to an article in *Journal of the American Medical Association* (June 14, 1990), a hospital study of 1,033 patients found 54 percent were low in magnesium. They reported that many of these patients died of magnesium deficiency–related symptoms.

demand more and more food until it gets what it needs. People who come to see me for a nutritional consultation are often embarrassed that they have no will power to stop eating. I tell them that once they feed their bodies nutrient-dense foods, they will be satisfied with less and their cravings will disappear. It works every time.

One finding of the U.S. Department of Agriculture's most recent (2006) National Health and Nutrition Examination Survey was that individuals eating a Standard American Diet lacked these seven important nutrients:

- Vitamin E: A fat-soluble vitamin found in some fats and oils and many foods, vitamin E is an antioxidant that helps to protect your cells from free radical damage. It also helps reduce damage to your body by environmental pollution and toxic chemicals. Foods that are high in vitamin E include: cold-pressed oils, organic eggs, molasses, leafy green vegetables, nuts and seeds, and organ meats.

- Magnesium: Of all the minerals, this one is crucial for good health. Unfortunately, industrial farming has stripped it from the soil, so you need to get it from organic food or supplements. It is essential for utilizing calcium properly, keeps your blood circulating smoothly, strengthens your heart, and calms your nerves. Foods that are high in magnesium are: leafy greens, pumpkin seeds, cucumbers, black and navy beans, nuts, whole grains, and tofu.

Healthy Tidbits

The percentage of magnesium that is lost during food processing is astounding:
- Refining of flour from wheat: 80%
- Polishing of rice: 83%
- Production of starch from corn: 97%
- Extraction of white sugar from molasses: 99%

- Calcium: Despite Americans consuming the highest amount of dairy products, we have the highest rates of osteoporosis in the world. This is due to the lack of magnesium in our diets. To better absorb calcium you need the proper ratio of magnesium. Calcium builds strong bones, supports muscle function, balances blood pressure, and calms your nerves. Sea vegetables are a huge source, as are green leafy vegetables, yogurt, asparagus, shellfish, molasses, and bone meal.

- Potassium: This important mineral works in sync with the dynamic duo, calcium and magnesium, to keep your panic attacks under control and prevent late-night leg cramps and twitching muscles. Most of all, it regulates your body fluids so your ankles won't swell on hot days. Best sources are whole grains, lean meats, vegetables, dried fruits, sunflower seeds, and bananas.

- Vitamin C: Here is your immune system booster and free radical fighter. You want this one to protect you against cancer and, hallelujah, slow down the aging process. Red foods like strawberries and red peppers are high in vitamin C, as are citrus fruits, cantaloupe, broccoli, cauliflower, and tomatoes.

- Vitamin A: This vitamin tends to get bad press due to warnings of taking too much. Not getting enough, however, can affect your eyesight, clear skin, and immune function. Don't leave home without it. The beta-carotene in carrots gives you a good dose of vitamin A, as do sweet potatoes, kale, spinach, apricots, and quality cod liver oil.

- Fiber: This is what helps you eliminate what you have eaten. Getting enough fiber will prevent constipation, help regulate cholesterol and blood sugar levels, and keep your weight down and your appetite satisfied. Yeah, baby. Whole grains, fresh fruits and vegetables, beans, and flaxseed meal are what you need to keep your bowels moving.

If we extend that list a bit further, my choice for most lacked nutrients would include:

- Omega-3 fatty acids: Your brain food, mood food, blood pressure valve and blood cleaner, omega-3 fatty acids must enter your body via food because your body does not make it on its own. Good old cod liver oil, like Grandma used to take, is the long-chain fatty acid, while flax, hemp, pumpkin, and chia seed oils are short-chain fatty acids. You want both in your diet. If your memory is fading, you suffer from depression, or are ADD/ADHD, then you for sure want to be taking the essential fatty acids. Omega-3 fatty acids can be taken in capsule form, by the tablespoon (flavored for taste appeal), or by eating plenty of clean fish, such as wild-caught salmon and cod.

- Vitamin D: This is the sunshine vitamin that we are not getting because we cover our skin with sun block. The sun's rays are important to your survival and are not necessarily the cause of skin cancer. By exposing your hands or arms to early-morning or late-afternoon sunlight for 20 to 30 minutes a day, you can absorb vitamin D. This can prevent depression, diabetes, osteoporosis, and breast and prostate cancer. Really, the list goes on and on. You can also get your vitamin D from eating fatty fish like salmon or cod and taking fish oil capsules. But the sun … now, that's the real source.

I hope you noticed that these essential vitamins, minerals, and nutrients come from whole, unrefined grains, vegetables, fruits, legumes, seeds, nuts, and some animal protein.

You are simply raising the quality of your food to the highest ingredients available. Eating this way will show you just how good you can feel all the time. You will be getting the nutrients essential for your body to function properly. I happen to know the end of the detox story and repeatedly have found it to be a very happy ending indeed.

> **Pure Insights** _____
>
> We are living in strange times when 784,000 people die annually from medical interventions yet many years go by and not one person dies as a result of taking supplements. Supplements decrease the cost of health care, and are essential for the prevention and treatment of a host of diseases.
>
> —Carolyn Dean, M.D., *Death By Modern Medicine*

What About Medications?

If you are currently taking pharmaceutical medications, make sure to have your doctor monitor your drug levels as your liver cleanses and your blood purifies. During the detox program your blood pressure and cholesterol levels may come down, your sinus infection can clear, your arthritic pains might ease, and your mood could brighten. The medications you are taking for these conditions will need to be altered or eliminated to reflect what is happening in your body.

When you take the time to detoxify your body and eat a whole-foods diet, you are taking responsibility for your own health. Once you begin to feel physically lighter, more energized, and mentally sharp, you have taken the first steps toward living a drug-free life. Congratulations, you may have just saved your own life!

Vitamins and Minerals

Supplements are an amalgam of concentrates and extracts that have been bound together in the lab by human hands hoping to come up with a balanced nutritional source of vitamins and minerals. It is best to first build the individual with good food, along with vitamin and mineral supplements. A building protocol can look like this:

- A supplement with iron for menstruating women
- A supplement without iron for nonmenstruating women
- Antioxidants, for the anti-aging factor
- Trace mineral tablet
- Omega-3 fatty acids
- B-complex, 50 milligrams
- Vitamin C, 500 milligrams
- Calcium, 1200 milligrams
- Magnesium, 400 milligrams

Healthy Tidbits

O blood types need L carnitine and B12 when lacking meat in their diet.

During the five-week detox program, you can follow this protocol for weeks one, two, four, and five. During week three, you will be fasting and won't need to take the supplements. Chapter 7 outlines particular herbs you can take during the cleansing phase of your detox and how they work.

If you are loath to taking a handful of pills, then consider taking a good food-grade daily multivitamin that provides all the essential vitamins and minerals. There are also liquid food supplements to drink in place of taking pills. As always, read labels carefully and consult your doctor or a licensed nutritionist before spending your money.

Supercleansing Foods

Foods you will want to eat on a regular basis are those that contribute to the strengthening of your immune system. They provide important nutrients along with taste to help reduce sweet cravings. The amount of sugar you consume can cause *glycation*, discovered to be the main factor in the aging process.

def•i•ni•tion

Glycation is a biochemical reaction that occurs in the body after a person consumes refined sugar and sugar-laden products. It is thought to be the main factor in the aging process.

Include the following list of superfoods in your daily diet as much as possible:

- Almonds: Shown to reduce total cholesterol. Useful source of calcium, and thought to build up a person's intellectual, spiritual, and reproductive abilities.

- Apples: Lowers cholesterol, removes heavy metals from the body, and helps to cleanse the liver and kidneys.

- Artichokes: Diuretic effect on the kidneys while helping to cleanse the liver of toxins. Helps to restore and promote the flow of bile from the gallbladder for better digestion of fats.

- Asparagus: A natural cleanser due to its diuretic properties. Helps to purge the results of sweet, refined, and intoxicating foods from the system.

- Berries: High in vitamin C and bioflavanoids. Some help to cleanse the liver, treat urinary tract infections, and correct disorders of the spleen and pancreas.

- Broccoli: High in phytonutrients and iron. With cleansing diuretic properties, it is considered to be the number-one cancer-fighting vegetable.

- Brown rice: Helps to cleanse the intestines by providing fiber. Used to treat the nervous system and treat depression. Good source of potassium and magnesium.

- Carrots: Helpful for stimulating the elimination of wastes by moving putrefactive bacteria out of the intestines. Rich source of beta-carotene. Absorbs and subdues free radicals in the body.

- Cranberries: Powerful antibacterial properties to help cleanse the kidneys, bladder, and urinary tract.

- Dandelions: Good source of iron and copper. Diuretic properties help in the treatment of high blood pressure and water retention. Cleansing and strengthening for the liver.

- Fennel: Supports weight loss by reducing water retention. Helps the body eliminate fats.

- Flaxseed: Good source of omega-3 fatty acids. Helps to thin the blood, reduce blood clotting. Cleanses the digestive tract, helping to prevent constipation. Helpful with weight loss. Grind the seeds and eat raw.

- Garlic: A natural antibiotic, promotes circulation and inhibits viral infections. An antidote to numerous ailments, it is antifungal, antibacterial, antiviral, and has been shown to lower blood pressure and rid the intestines of parasites.

For detox purposes eating garlic will support the development of the natural bacterial flora while killing pathogenic organisms in your digestive tract. Make this member of the onion, shallot, and leek family a tasty addition to many of your favorite recipes.

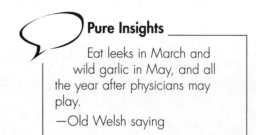

Pure Insights

Eat leeks in March and wild garlic in May, and all the year after physicians may play.
—Old Welsh saying

♦ Ginger: Has a warming and stimulating effect on the body. Good for nausea, diarrhea, and bloating. Nutritionally supports the digestive process and has the ability to help settle the stomach. Studies show ginger is as effective as over-the-counter medications in helping to prevent motion sickness. For detox purposes ginger can be eaten or taken as a tea daily.

♦ Kale: High in the nutrients iron, beta-carotene, and calcium. Used to ease lung congestion and stimulate the immune system.

♦ Lemons: Alkalinizes the blood, helps to cleanse the liver by stimulating the release of enzymes.

♦ Onions: Antivirus properties, high in antioxidants, good for clearing the lungs.

♦ Pumpkin seeds: Good source of zinc, iron, and selenium. Helps in decreasing inflammation of the skin.

♦ Quinoa: High in protein, gluten-free so easy to digest, quick to cook, and a good source of vitamins and minerals.

♦ Radishes: Excellent detoxifier! Clears heavy mucus from the sinuses, throat, and lungs. Relieves indigestion and bloating. Eliminates food stagnation in the digestive tract. One tablespoon of grated radish taken daily for two or three weeks helps treat gallstones, kidney stones, and bladder stones. Serve it in a salad or grated and tossed with some apple cider vinegar.

♦ Salad greens: High in natural enzymes and antioxidants. Helps to cleanse the digestive tract.

♦ Sea vegetables: High source of calcium and minerals. Alkalinizes the blood, helps to clean the lymphatic system, and relieves swelling in the body. Easy to prepare, but requires presoaking. Use wakame in miso soup, nori to wrap your rice and veggies, or arame tossed into a vegetable stir-fry.

♦ Sesame seeds: High in iron and calcium. Black sesame seeds are used to lubricate the heart, liver, kidneys, pancreas, and lungs. Contains excellent laxative properties for detoxifying the colon.

> **Pure Insights** _____
>
> Let food be your medicine and medicine your food.
>
> —Hippocrates

♦ Shiitake mushrooms: A prized cancer fighter, shiitakes help to discharge accumulated fat and cholesterol in the blood. They are a good source of germanium, an element that strengthens your immune system and improves cellular oxygenation. Delicious sautéed with onions and served over your favorite burger.

♦ Tomatoes (in season): Cleans the liver, alkalizes the blood, and is a rich source of lycopene, which protects against heart disease and cancer.

♦ Walnuts: Good source of omega-3 fatty acids and a cholesterol-lowering food. Also a good source of copper to support immune function, while walnut kernels are used to help in healing inflammatory skin conditions such as eczema.

♦ Watercress: Contains strong diuretic properties and is a good blood purifier.

Green Foods

Green foods have been scientifically proven to have health benefits for the body and mind. There are five excellent sources of green foods:

♦ Chlorella

♦ Spirulina

♦ Wheat grass

♦ Barley grass

♦ Blue green algae

They are all excellent sources of two important phytochemicals, chlorophyll and lycopene. Compared with the other four, chlorella boasts the highest chlorophyll content. These powerful foods have the outstanding ability to eliminate toxins, pesticides, and heavy metals from the body.

Green foods are considered complete foods and an easily assimilated source of nutrients. They are regarded as a superior source of vitamins and minerals compared to regular dietary supplements. As always, nature does it better. The health benefits of green foods are as follows:

- Strengthen your immune system
- Detoxify heavy metals and pesticides
- Improve your digestion
- Improve your elimination
- Improve mental focus
- Increase and sustain your energy level
- Alkalinize your blood pH

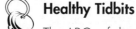

Healthy Tidbits

The ABCs of detoxing and healing your body are activate, build, and cleanse. Activate is your commitment to take responsibility for your own health by natural means. Build is to strengthen and support the immune system. Cleansing allows your filtering organs to eliminate any toxins, chemicals, and poisons.

Green foods come in capsule or powder form. Look for a blend that is certified organic. There are also blends providing four to six servings of concentrated fruits, vegetables, and sprouted whole grains along with the microalgaes. Although this may not seem very appetizing, you can improve on the taste by mixing the powder in your morning smoothie.

Protein and Meal Powders

Protein powders are a highly concentrated form of protein made from soy, whey, egg, rice, pea, hemp, or sprouted grains. In the first two weeks you can use a dairy- and soy-free protein in your morning smoothies, or add it to baked goods when making breakfast muffins or cookies.

The hemp seed provides high amounts of sustainable protein in an easily digested form. Try not to make your protein source a processed powder. It is better to grind your own seeds for freshness and maximum nutrient content. It is a good alternative to a powdered protein.

There are also some excellent meal powders made up of a mixture of sprouted grains, vegetables, green foods, and fruits. These provide a nutrient-dense food in powder form that is best combined with fruit or vegetable juice and mixed in a blender. Look for brands that contain organic, raw, and sprouted ingredients.

Flaxseed Meal

High in omega-3 fatty acids, flaxseed meal should become a regular part of your diet. Try adding a tablespoon to your morning smoothie, cooked grains, and baked goods.

Because the body cannot manufacture this necessary fatty acid, it must be provided in your daily diet. The Standard American Diet has an overabundance of omega-6 fatty acids and not enough omega-3.

When in balance, these two fatty acids are essential for regulating the cardiovascular, immune, digestive, and reproductive systems; they control inflammation and healing; and they support the functions of the brain, your body thermostat, and how your body burns calories.

Flaxseed meal provides the highest amount of short-chain fatty acids, while fish oil is the best source of long-chain fatty acids. Flaxseed oil should never be heated, but taken in its raw state and kept refrigerated.

> **Pure Insights** _____
>
>   Although it has been used therapeutically for over 5,000 years, only recently have scientists learned that flaxseed may lower blood cholesterol levels, that are often associated with heart attacks and strokes, reduce the viscosity of blood, lower arterial blood pressure, prevent colon and breast cancer, improve moods, diminish allergies and produce healthier skin.
>
> —James R. Johnston, *Flaxseed (Linseed) Oil and the Power of Omega-3*

Try including 1 to 2 tablespoons of flaxseed meal a day when making the transition from a low-fiber to a high-fiber diet. You may experience some digestive irritation in the form of intestinal gas and possible cramping for the first day or two. It will help to drink an extra glass of water. Flaxseed absorbs eight times its weight in water, which makes it an excellent bulking agent. This will help you maintain bowel regularity and support your body in the process of losing weight.

Probiotics

In Chapter 4, I wrote about how yeast and parasites can take over your colon unless you replant the good microflora into your intestines. With this in mind, you should take three essential *probiotics* during your detox: acidophilus, bifidus, and L. reuteri.

Our "roots" are our intestinal tract, where we absorb water and nutrients. Bacteria play an important role in our "root" system. There are 3 to 4 pounds of friendly microorganisms living in our intestinal tract, most of them bacteria. You want to be sure to take live probiotics morning and evening to help replant the intestinal flora, while minimizing the expansion of yeast and parasites. When purchasing probiotics from a health-food store, look for refrigerated brands containing 8 to 14 billion live cells per capsule. It's best if the label says the cells are live at the end of expiration rather than at the time of manufacture.

def•i•ni•tion

Probiotics means "pro life," while antibiotics means "against life." As beneficial as antibiotics have proven to be against bacterial infections, they are also powerful destroyers of the good intestinal flora in your gut. This friendly flora promotes the body's natural immunity, aids in digesting your food, and generally keeps you strong and healthy.

The Least You Need to Know

◆ The experience of detoxing your body can be a time of physical change, mental reflection, and personal transformation.

◆ Your protein intake should make up about 15 to 20 percent of your daily calories, which means 4 ounces (the size of a deck of cards) per meal.

◆ The whole purpose of eating food is to provide nutrient sustenance to your body; most Americans are eating foods that are lacking crucial vitamins and minerals.

◆ Foods you will want to eat on a regular basis are those that contribute to the strengthening of your immune system and provide important nutrients for the entire body.

◆ Green foods are considered complete foods, an easily assimilated source of nutrients, and a superior source of vitamins and minerals compared to regular dietary supplements.

◆ There are 3 or 4 pounds of friendly microorganisms living in your intestinal tract, most of them a form of bacteria you can replace by taking probiotics.

Moving the Process Along

In This Chapter

- ◆ Nature's herbal helpers
- ◆ Should you use laxatives?
- ◆ The best detox herbs
- ◆ Other cleansing supplements
- ◆ Fiber to the rescue
- ◆ Washing away the debris

In the natural world, nature has provided an antidote for all that might ail the human race. We are inextricably connected to all things on Earth, and they to us. Plants, soil, air, and water help us to survive and stay healthy. We make our medicines from them, cleanse our bodies with them, and find our nutrition through them. It is fitting, then, that we use what Mother Nature has given us to detoxify our organs in a gentle, natural way.

In this chapter, you will find plants, herbs, and Earth products that work synergistically with your body. Provided by Mother Nature and available in your natural foods market, they help you to go deeper and be more effective in detoxing your body.

Nature's Pharmacopeia

Herbs have always been used to heal, regenerate, activate, create, soothe, calm, excite, and cleanse the human body. They have a unique quality, and some say each individual plant has an energetic spirit. It is this energy, as much as it is the healing properties of the plant, that works synergistically with your energy.

As medicine, herbs are body balancers. They work with your body's many systems as foundation nutrients. Do not expect herbs to act the same way that drugs do. Pharmaceutical drugs are designed to treat the symptom of an illness and require an increase in the dosage over time to get the same effect. Herbs, on the other hand, gently penetrate into your body's organs, tissues, and glands. This takes a bit more time before you will see results.

In *Elementary Treatise in Herbology* (1978), Dr. Edward E. Shook wrote: "Modern science now comes to our assistance and through chemical analysis reveals the fact that all the chemical element's of which our bodies are composed, are contained in the roots, barks, leaves, flowers and fruits of Herbs. Each family of plants has its own peculiar habit of taking from the soil a specific group of chemical elements."

You could say that herbs are food in a concentrated form. This gives them the unique ability to address both the symptoms and causes of an illness. Herbs provide nutrients that may otherwise be lacking in the diet due to the processing and contamination of our food, soil, and air. As food, most herbs are safe to eat and often enhance a recipe with their particular flavor. Many of the common foods and herbs you use in cooking are known for their medicinal qualities:

- ◆ Parsley: A good diuretic that helps to flush the kidneys of toxins. Rich in anti-oxidants, parsley supports and strengthens the liver. It is high in chlorophyll, making it an excellent blood cleanser. It is a good source of calcium, thiamine, riboflavin, potassium, iron, vitamin C, vitamin A, niacin, phosphorus, sulphur, magnesium, and silicon. Add it to salads, as a topping for pasta, on fish or chicken, and in pesto. Parsley is also effective in helping to reduce the lingering smell of garlic on the breath.

- ◆ Capsicum: Your hot and spicy addition to recipes, it is often added to many herbal formulas as a catalyst for the other herbs. Its red color is partly due to its high vitamin A content. Capsicum influences blood flow, which makes it food for the circulatory system. It helps to reduce inflammation of the joints and expel excess mucus from the body. You will find it used in the lemonade master cleanse recipe (see Chapter 11) for this purpose.

◆ Sage: The herb you use in your holiday stuffing is a member of the mint family. Its name comes from the Latin *salvare*, which means "to heal." It has antioxidant properties and has been used as a preservative for centuries. Native Americans cleanse the energy of a space or a person by burning sage. Its aromatic properties help sage create an environment that is unfriendly to foreign invaders, both physically and spiritually.

◆ Dandelion: A member of the sunflower family, it is considered by herbalists to be one of the most nutrient-rich foods in the plant kingdom. The reason being that the whole plant is edible—the flowers, the leaves, the roots. It's a very powerful diuretic and one of the best natural sources of potassium. The dandelion root is prescribed by herbalists for inflammation and congestion of the liver and gallbladder. This amazing green superfood is a source of potassium, calcium, iron, manganese, magnesium, silicon, phosphorus, and sodium. The leaves are a richer source of vitamin A than carrots and contain vitamins B, C, and D.

> **Healthy Tidbits**
>
> Dandelion flowers make an excellent liver tonic. In the springtime gather a bowl full of unsprayed dandelion flower tops and pour 4 cups of boiling water over them. Cover with a clean cloth and allow to steep for four hours. Strain and sweeten. Sip warm or chilled throughout the spring days.

◆ Green tea: Helps fight damaging free radicals because it is rich in bioflavonoid compounds. It helps to support your immune and circulatory systems, possesses antimicrobial properties, and helps normalize vascular blood clotting and total cholesterol. For detox purposes drink 2 to 3 cups a day to support healthy kidney function.

According to Jeffrey Blumberg, Ph.D., of Tufts University in Boston, Oriental teas may play an important role in helping to prevent heart disease and cancer. Tea contains a variety of phytochemicals, including polyphenols and flavonoids. Acting as antioxidants, they kill free radicals that might otherwise damage the body's cell membranes and lead to a variety of chronic diseases.

Try to include these amazing foods in your detox program on a daily or weekly basis. Check the menu suggestions in Chapters 9 through 13 for ideas on how to use them (see Appendix B for additional recipes).

Using Herbal Laxatives

Laxatives have been commonly used for constipation, as far back as the fourth century B.C.E. At that time in Greece, Hippocrates, the father of medicine, was developing his Humoral theory. This was based on maintaining equilibrium between what he called the four humors: blood, phlegm, yellow bile, and black bile. Laxatives were used to purge the bowels of poisons and restore the body's natural equilibrium. Then, as now, natural herbs and oils were used for their laxative properties, along with eating plenty of high-fiber foods.

def•i•ni•tion

The word **laxative** is derived from the Latin word *laxus,* which means "loose." Laxatives are substances that stimulate defecation and aid in the smooth transit of fecal material through the gastrointestinal tract.

Herbal laxatives can be used to regenerate a sluggish and constipated colon, or they can calm a spastic colon subject to uncontrolled diarrhea. Mother Nature has provided an antidote for this difficulty.

A sluggish colon is a buildup of putrid waste products, causing a backup in the large intestine. Symptoms are constipation, gas, bad breath, headaches, skin problems, and fatigue.

A spastic colon (colitis) is too much peristalsis or muscular tightness in the bowels. Symptoms are diarrhea, gas, and bloating.

Healthy Tidbits

Diarrhea alternating with constipation is most likely poor digestion and/or a spastic colon. For this condition, add slippery elm bark and begin with 500 milligrams of magnesium, going as high as 1000 until you find relief. Eating soft, cooked brown rice can also help.

Diarrhea is a sign that your colon is trying to eliminate toxic irritants. You will want to treat this with fiber foods like psyllium seed and slippery elm bark, which help to absorb and eliminate the toxins. Probiotics are essential for both treating and preventing diarrhea; however, in the case of severe diarrhea, see your doctor, as the threat of dehydration should not be ignored.

Constipation requires more stimulating laxatives, but treat them with the respect they deserve. For example, cascara sagrada is a stronger-acting laxative than senna, and is best used for flaccid bowels and chronic constipation. Used in this manner, for a short period of time, this stimulating herb can help train the intestinal muscles to work again.

Laxatives should be taken only when needed and under the supervision of an experienced health practitioner. They are not to be used as a weight-loss tool. Used medicinally, they can retrain your intestinal muscles to work properly. Take too many for too long, and you build up a dependency. As always, moderation is the key.

Cleansing Herbal Supplements

Herbs known for cleansing your organs pave the way for the body to do its own work. Herbs used for detoxing purposes break up toxins, cleanse organs and glands, lubricate, tone, and nourish the digestive system. The list of herbs is many and varied. Body detox kits can be found in your health-food store, but which ones should you buy? Your five-week detox program is a food-based detoxification, but using herbal supplements can enhance your efforts.

Slippery Elm Bark

Slippery elm bark comes from a deciduous tree native to the United States and Canada. The inner bark of the slippery elm was used widely by the Native Americans and later by the early American settlers to ease digestive discomfort.

Slippery elm bark is perfect for your detox program, and its benefits are legendary:

◆ Supports healthy digestion

◆ Soothes the digestive tract

◆ Helps maintain normal elimination

◆ Absorbs toxins from the bowel

◆ Provides *mucilage* to soothe the digestive tract

◆ Helps relieve throat and digestive discomfort

◆ Supports your body during convalescence

◆ Relieves skin irritation

def•i•ni•tion

Mucilage is a long chain of sugars (polysaccharides) that make a slippery substance when combined with water. It can settle the digestive tract, absorb toxins from the bowel, and help maintain regular bowel elimination.

Slippery elm bark is rich in nutrients, easy to digest, and soothing to the digestive system, making it an excellent food during times of digestive discomfort. It can be made into a gruel, but know that it quickly expands when added to water. During your detox, you can take slippery elm bark in capsule, bulk, or tea form to help absorb toxins and maintain waste elimination. It also helps to relieve gas and bloating and provides mucilage to soothe irritated or inflamed intestinal tissue.

An Herbal "Master List" for Detoxing

Herbs work best in combination with other herbs, because they can be formulated to reach several parts of the body at once. Here is an example of 22 herbs synergistically combined to support proper digestion and waste elimination. This formula supports and promotes the proper functioning of the liver, colon, and kidneys; aids digestion; and acts as a cleansing agent for the major detoxifying organs. When buying an herbal formula, look for one that contains all or most of these herbs. The recommended dosage is to take two capsules with a meal three times daily, and drink plenty of water throughout the day.

This formula contains the herb cascara sagrada. For a milder laxative, use a combination containing the herb senna.

1. Gentian root: Stomach tonic

2. Irish moss: Soothes inflamed tissues

3. Cascara sagrada bark: Laxative

4. Fenugreek seeds: Expels toxic waste

5. Golden seal root: Anti-inflammatory

6. Slippery elm bark: Soothes stomach and digestive tract

7. Safflower flower: Clears liver and gallbladder

8. Black walnut hulls: Kills parasites

9. Myrrh gum: Cleans and soothes the intestines

10. Parthenium root: Immune booster and diuretic

11. Yellow dock root: Blood purifier and builder

12. Dandelion root: Detoxifies poisons from the liver

13. Oregon grape root and rhizome: Blood cleanser

14. Uva ursi leaf extract: Strengthens bladder and kidneys

15. Chickweed leaf extract: Treats blood toxicity

16. Catnip herb: Calms the nervous system

17. Cyani flower: Treats inflammation and infections

18. Cilantro: Effective in removing heavy metals

19. Burdock root: Blood purifier

20. Marshmellow root: Removes excess mucus

21. Milk thistle: Removes drug residue from the liver

22. Thyme: Kills yeast overgrowth

 Detox Alert _____

Before taking any herbal supplement, see your health-care provider, especially if pregnant or nursing, any medical condition exists, or when taking any medications. Read and follow recommendations carefully.

Activated Charcoal

Activated charcoal is used to detoxify the intestines because it absorbs irritants in the digestive tract. As an absorbent, it is useful for treating diarrhea, intestinal gas, indigestion, and poisons. It has the appearance of fine black powder. It is a type of carbon made from wood, vegetables, and other materials. It has been found to lower total cholesterol, especially the bad LDL cholesterol. Activated charcoal has absorbent, antidiarrheal, antidote, antitoxic, and antivenomous properties.

People use activated charcoal for bloating, bad-smelling gas, high cholesterol, poison or drug overdose, and detoxification purposes.

It is useful to know that it is used for water filtration and works in a similar way in your digestive system. When activated charcoal is ingested it passes into the intestines, attracting organic chemicals which bond to the charcoal, allowing them to be eliminated.

Detox Alert _____

Do not take activated charcoal with prescription medications and nutritional supplements, as it can interfere with their assimilation and effectiveness. It's a good idea to check with your doctor before taking this or any supplement.

Buy it in capsule form and use two capsules with meals at the first sign of intestinal gas or distress. You can take activated charcoal for a short time then discontinue its use. The first week of your detox program, take six to eight capsules a day.

For detoxification purposes, more is not necessarily better, and activated charcoal can cause constipation if taken in large doses. Drink plenty of water when taking this supplement.

Don't be concerned if taking activated charcoal turns your stools black. Although there haven't been adverse effects in amounts used in nutritional supplements, there are no studies on the long-term safety of activated charcoal in humans. Pregnant or nursing women and the elderly should avoid activated charcoal.

Bentonite Clay

Here is another natural product you can use to absorb toxins, chemicals, and poisons from your bowels. Basically, it is sedimentary clay composed of weathered and aged volcanic ash. Now, it may seem unusual to ingest clay, but then this isn't any ordinary clay. When *bentonite* becomes hydrated, the electrical and molecular components of the clay rapidly change and produce an "electrical charge." This charge gives the clay its ability to absorb toxins, impurities, heavy metals, and other internal contaminants.

def•i•ni•tion

Bentonite is sedimentary clay composed of weathered and aged volcanic ash. The largest and most active deposits are found in Wyoming and Montana. When mixed with water, it rapidly swells open like a highly porous sponge. The toxins are drawn into the sponge through electrical attraction, and once there they are bound within the clay.

Bentonite clay's structure attracts and soaks up toxins on its exterior wall, then slowly draws them into the interior center of the clay where they are held in a sort of repository. Combining the use of bentonite clay with the appropriate herbal supplements and lots of water helps eliminate any poisons from the body via the large intestines.

Bentonite clay is mined from deep within the earth. Superior-quality clay comes from vital and healthy land chosen for the proper characteristics and consistency required of edible clay. Once it has been brought out into the sunlight, it is dried and then granulated with huge crushers. It is then inspected by a quality-control team and packaged for your use.

You can find bentonite clay in capsule form and in cleansing kits, which will make it easier to determine proper amounts. These kits will also provide the necessary herbs to stimulate the removal of the clay from your digestive system.

Digestive Enzymes

Digestive enzymes are proteins crucial for breaking down foods into nutrients your body can absorb. Normally you produce about 22 different digestive enzymes, but age and stress reduce this amount. In addition, you tax your body by not chewing your food properly. Mastication of food in the mouth releases the enzymes needed for proper digestion. Without enzymes, vitamins would be useless.

When you eat a meal, digestive enzymes that are released from your salivary glands, stomach, and small intestine immediately get to work to speed up the digestive process. Each enzyme acts on a specific type of food. Protease, for example, breaks down the components of protein. Amylase helps digest carbohydrates; lipase breaks down fats; and cellulose, found in plants, digests fiber.

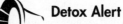 **Detox Alert**

Bloating, gas, heartburn, and indigestion are common signs of poor digestion. You don't have to wait until you have symptoms to take enzymes. In the absence of symptoms, enzymes help maintain optimal digestion and absorption of the vital nutrients in food.

The strength of our immune system is dependant on the amount of enzyme reserves we have. White blood cells and enzymes work together to destroy foreign, disease-causing substances in the blood and lymph fluid. Using all your enzymes for digestion leaves your immune system fighting alone.

Due to malnutrition, over-refined foods, environmental toxins, and poor health, many people are lacking these important enzymes. During the five-week detox program, take one or two digestive enzymes with each meal and snack.

For other purposes, such as skin inflammation, doctors recommend taking digestive enzyme supplements on an empty stomach. Enzymes not used to digest a meal seem to gravitate to areas of inflammation in the body where they help digest foreign matter that may be causing allergic reactions.

The Benefits of Fiber

Although dietary fiber is considered to have laxative effects, it is not a laxative. It is, however, the first step in dealing with constipation. Because fiber moves through your bowels at a normal rate, it acts as an internal regulator, making elimination smooth and easy. Laxatives, on the other hand, speed-skate through your bowels, pushing forward everything in their way.

Healthy Tidbits _____

Adult-onset diabetes can be successfully treated with high dietary fiber, and those taking insulin can often reduce their requirements by adhering to a fiber-rich diet.

According to the National Academy of Sciences' Institute of Medicine, the intake of dietary fiber for an adult should be between 21 and 38 grams per day. Most Americans consume an average of 14 to 15 grams per day, much less than is recommended. In the senior population fiber intake is found to be even lower, and a fiber supplement is often required to improve bowel function.

Dietary fiber is classified as soluble and insoluble, each having unique health benefits. Soluble fiber can help to lower blood cholesterol levels and can be found in oat bran, oatmeal, barley, fruits, peas, and beans. Plantago psyllium is a soluble fiber product used as a bulking and lubricating agent for the digestive system. All parts of the plant are used by some cultures, but the seed and seed hulls are preferred. You can take it in capsule form or use a teaspoon full in water upon rising in the morning.

Insoluble fibers increase overall stool volume and stimulate normal bowel contractions, thus reducing transit time through the colon. Apart from their laxative effect, insoluble fibers have been shown to prevent the symptoms associated with conditions such as irritable bowel syndrome and diverticulitis. Insoluble fibers can be found in apples, broccoli, cabbage, corn, carrots, and potatoes.

Fiber is a key component of fruits, vegetables, nuts, seeds, legumes, and whole grains. Despite the tough chew you can get with animal flesh, it is not considered fiber food. Fiber should be added slowly to your diet, and to avoid constipation be sure to drink six to eight glasses of water each day.

Internal Water Cleansing

Internal water cleansing, also called colon hydrotherapy, is a method of gently washing your large intestine, removing accumulated fecal matter, mucus, harmful toxins, and bacteria from the bowel. Your colon is a four-layer muscle, and like any muscle, if it is not toned and working efficiently, it becomes slow and flaccid. The process of colon hydrotherapy helps to stimulate and exercise this muscle.

The health of your colon determines the health of your organs, along with the nervous, circulatory, endocrine, digestive, muscular, lymphatic, reproductive, skeletal, urinary, respiratory, and immune systems of your body. Where waste material accumulates over years and years, it can become stagnant and toxic. If you are constipated and not eliminating daily, then your colon is not working properly. Waste and toxins that remain too long in the intestines feed harmful bacteria, causing putrefaction and fermentation, which in turn can cause symptoms such as gas, bloating, headaches, fatigue, and skin problems. These poisons can also be reabsorbed into the system and cause auto-intoxification or self-poisoning, and can lead to more serious health problems.

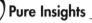

> **Pure Insights**
>
> The very best of diets can be no better than the very worst, if the sewage system of the colon is clogged with a collection of waste and corruption.
> —Norman Walker, Ph.D.

At any time throughout the five-week detox program, consult your doctor about doing a series of colon hydrotherapy sessions. The treatment consists of a gentle infusion of filtered, temperature-controlled water into the colon, by way of a sterile-disposable rectal tube or speculum. It is a very simple process that moves clean water into the colon/large intestine, in order to flush out fecal matter.

There is some speculation in the medical field that colonics are safe and/or necessary. If you are considering having this done, you will need to see an experienced certified colon hydrotherapist. The process can be safe and effective under the guidance of a licensed professional. Make sure the professional uses FDA-approved equipment and disposable rectal speculums, and follows proper sterilizing procedures. Colonics are not a requirement of the detox program, but one option that some may wish to pursue.

The Least You Need to Know

- The energetic spirits of individual herbs are used to heal, regenerate, activate, create, soothe, calm, excite, and cleanse the human body.

- Herbal laxatives can be used to regenerate a sluggish and constipated colon, or they can calm a spastic colon subject to uncontrolled diarrhea.

- Herbs used for detoxification purposes break up toxins; cleanse organs and glands; and lubricate, tone, and nourish the digestive system.

- Activated charcoal is used to detoxify the intestines because it absorbs irritants in the digestive tract, and is useful for treating diarrhea, intestinal gas, indigestion, and poisons.

- Normally you produce about 22 different digestive enzymes, which are proteins crucial for breaking down foods into nutrients your body can absorb.

- Colon hydrotherapy is a method of gently washing your large intestine, which removes accumulated fecal matter, mucus, harmful toxins, and bacteria from the bowel.

Chapter **8**

Detox Side Effects

In This Chapter

- The "die-off" effect
- Feeling worse before you feel better
- What your body is telling you
- Relieving detox symptoms
- Past health problems revisited
- Medical treatments that can help

If your organs are overloaded with toxins, chemicals, pharmaceutical, and/ or recreational drugs, it is possible you will experience a physical reaction while detoxifying. As they clean, your filtering organs will be dumping waste products into your bloodstream and intestines, out through the pores of your skin and possibly your nasal passages. Then again, that may not happen if you are following the guidelines in Chapters 9 through 13 and taking the transition process one step at a time.

In this chapter, you will discover the ingenious ways your body speaks to you, the cleansing reactions you may experience, and how to relieve these adverse reactions and go deeper into the detoxification process.

The Herxheimer Reaction

When your body is cleansing faster than it can eliminate toxins, you will experience Herxheimer's "die-off" reaction. A Herxheimer reaction is a healing crisis that occurs when the body is detoxifying too rapidly and toxins are being released faster than the body can eliminate them. This reaction was first documented by Jarisch Adolf Herxheimer, an Austrian dermatologist. In collaboration with his brother Karl, they found that when treating their patients, many of them developed severe physical reactions to the treatments before shifting into a healing phase. The patients were usually very ill for two or three days, after which they began to feel better.

While following the five-week detox program, you can avoid this by changing your food and environment slowly. Your goal should be to make a smooth transition in a gradual and gentle manner.

The "die-off" reaction occurs when toxic microbes in your body are starved of the foods that feed them, such as sugar, dairy, and alcohol; or they are exposed to anti-microbial herbs, which kill them off. The cell-wall proteins of these microbes are absorbed through the body's weakened mucous membrane and eliminated. However, if this is happening too fast, there will be too many dead microbes in your system and you may experience uncomfortable symptoms.

When detoxifying, the body is responding to a change of diet as an opportunity to rid itself of toxins. Your filtering organs will take advantage of the small opening to do some needed house cleaning. That's why it is important to have time scheduled for yourself. You will need to step back from everything, rest, and let the detox proceed.

The Usual Detox Reactions

"You may feel worse before you feel better" is a holistic phrase referring to a process called *retracing*. This is a good sign that your body is responding properly but is overwhelmed with what is being released.

def•i•ni•tion

Retracing is when you feel worse as your organs detox, before you feel better.

As your body is eliminating toxins, it is also working to rebalance all its systems. Herxheimer reactions can mimic the symptoms you were experiencing before you began your detox:

◆ Headaches

◆ Flulike symptoms

- Diarrhea
- Muscle aches
- Joint pain
- Skin rash
- Fatigue
- Lymph node swelling
- Skin eruptions

- Nausea
- Sleepiness
- Constipation
- Head or chest cold
- Ear infections
- Boils

When a symptom appears and is suppressed with medications, it may disappear for a while, but will eventually return or show up as another kind of symptom. If a skin rash occurs, it can mean your body is working to eliminate toxins through the skin. If you try to suppress it with a topical steroid cream, it may clear but show up later as chronic diarrhea. We know this signals that your body is attempting to rid itself of toxins.

Sinus infections are a great example. Some people take five different medications for chronic sinus infections, which can also show up as bronchitis, ear infections, and constipation. Even with the medications, relief is minimal until milk, cheese, ice cream, and yogurt are eliminated from the diet. Once off the dairy, detoxify the colon, and the sinuses will clear and infections will be a thing of the past.

Detox Alert

When experiencing a Herxheimer reaction, it is important not to suppress these temporary symptoms with drugs, or the healing process may become interrupted.

If you experience an initial increase in urination, in bowel movements, or even spells of anxiety, you are not getting worse; you are actually getting better. Although everyone's reactions differ, eventually this will pass.

An initial healing crisis usually lasts around three days, but if your immunity is low, it may last a week or more. The severity of these reactions will vary from person to person depending on immune strength, bowel function, and how your organs of detoxification are working. If you had a diet heavy in red meats, for example, and become a vegetarian overnight, you might have severe symptoms for a time. If your lifestyle changes are as gradual as are outlined in Chapters 9 through 13, the symptoms could be less severe.

It may help to know that those uncomfortable symptoms indicate that your body is effectively eliminating any toxic substances.

Understanding Your Body's Language

Your body's unique intelligence has a way of telling you when something is wrong and it needs help. Not understanding this language makes it difficult to know when your body is talking to you. In Eastern medicine, a doctor will read what is written in your face, tongue, eyes, skin, and pulse. The signs of depletion are all there, and may have been for some time.

Visual diagnosis is an ancient tool used by traditional healers to discover the strengths, weaknesses, and health (or lack of health) within the body. Once awareness of what's happening inside the body becomes evident, it can be used to diagnose an illness or prevent an illness from fully manifesting. Awareness of your body is the key to figuring out the necessary diet and lifestyle adjustments to obtain vibrant health.

> **Pure Insights**
>
> If your body is in a state of vibrant health the skin glows, the eyes are bright and clear, the hair is healthy and nails strong. If the skin is uneven in tone and texture, the eyes are dull, lifeless or red with broken capillaries, and the hair and nails are brittle, dry, and weak, your body may be signaling to you that you need to cleanse your system. It's time to detox!
>
> —Andrea Beaman, holistic health counselor and author of *The Whole Truth Eating and Recipe Guide*

Facial diagnosis is based on the principle that, in utero, certain parts of your body were forming and strengthening at the same time as your facial features. According to this principle each area of your face manifests a corresponding organ and how it is functioning in the body:

- ◆ Your cheeks represent lungs and their condition.

- ◆ Tip of the nose is heart.

- ◆ Nostrils represent the bronchi of the lungs.

- ◆ Middle part of the nose is stomach.

- ◆ Upper part of the nose is pancreas.

- Under the eyes reflects your kidneys.

- Between the eyebrows shows liver condition.

- The temples reflect your spleen.

- Your forehead represents small intestines.

- Peripheral forehead shows the large intestine.

- Upper forehead is the bladder.

- Ears show kidney function.

- Your mouth reflects the condition of your entire digestive tract.

- Around the mouth indicates the condition of your sexual organs.

> **Pure Insights** _____
>
> Knowing is the beginning of freedom. The art of knowing is the art of realizing freedom. All suffering comes from ignorance: Ignorance of what I am, ignorance of who I am, of what we are. The art of knowing is the opening of the secret of life, and a path for health, happiness and eternal life.
>
> —Michio Kushi, *Book of Oriental Diagnosis*

You can easily apply these guidelines to your personal health:

- Women tend to break out under their lower lip when approaching their monthly menstruation.

- Gum and tooth infections are related to the condition of the intestines, and much of this can be resolved by detoxing these organs.

- Someone with a large bulbous nose shows their heart straining against clogged arteries.

- Swollen under-eyes reflect kidneys unable to work properly, and a retention of fluid from eating too much salt and fatty foods.

- The classic lines between the eyebrows show your liver working hard to keep up with your lifestyle.

- Yellowing of the whites of the eyes indicates liver jaundice.

Basically, the condition of your health is all right there, each morning, in front of your eyes. Your face never lies. It shows us when energy becomes blocked in any part of the body; it affects us both internally and externally. According to visual diagnosis every blemish, mole, and discoloration has a deeper meaning.

Relieving Symptoms

To counter these "die-off" reactions, your body needs fresh vegetable juices and a lot of water to help wash out the toxins. You want to eat potassium-rich foods, because you are losing this important mineral with excessive urination, diarrhea, and perspiration.

Potassium brings balance to your cells, clears out excess sodium, and is a great boost for inner cleansing. The Food and Nutrition Board of the National Academy of Sciences-National Research Council estimates that adults need 1,875 to 5,625 milligrams of potassium daily. This ensures that your heart receives what is essential to perform with regularity.

Make a pot of Potassium Broth and have a bowl or two during the day to help counter the Herxheimer reactions you are experiencing.

Potassium Broth

Makes 6 cups

1 cup celery, chopped

1 cup carrot, grated

$\frac{1}{2}$ cup watercress, chopped

1 quart water

1 cup tomatoes, chopped, seeds removed

2 red skinned potatoes, chopped

1 tsp. dried basil

Pinch of sea salt

Combine all ingredients in a heavy saucepan, bring to a boil, reduce heat and simmer for 30 minutes. Serve with toasted pumpkin seeds and a teaspoon of light miso (optional).

Other potassium-rich foods include bananas, dried apricots (sulfur-free), sprouts, seeds, and nuts. Play with some of these salad variations that are tasty and loaded with potassium:

◆ Apple, grated carrot, raisins, and walnuts sprinkled with cinnamon, lemon, and apple juice

- Red-and-white-cabbage slaw with toasted sunflower seeds and a thin coating of pesto mayonnaise (dairy-free)
- Assorted fresh sprouts, watercress, and arugula tossed with apple cider vinegar and extra-virgin olive oil

If you have a vegetable juicer, take it out of storage and try a few of these healthful combinations:

- Carrot, ginger, and apple
- Cucumber, carrot, parsley, and garlic
- Carrot, beet, and celery
- Beet (including greens) and carrot

You can also juice organic grapes and apples. Combine 1 cup of juice in a blender with half a banana, a few pitted dates, and a tablespoon of flax meal. Delicious!

A time-honored method of detoxification is to pour 8 ounces of boiling water over a few prunes (now called dried plums) and let them soften. Then eat the prunes and drink the water on an empty stomach. This potassium-rich fruit is also high in vitamin A. The combination melts the sludge in your colon, effectively eliminating it from your bowels.

Detox Alert

Mostly it is not the disease that kills you; it is the symptom of the disease that kills you. Treat the symptoms nutritionally. People die of the deficiencies the disease causes.

To help move the toxins out of your body more quickly, consider doing a series of colon hydrotherapy sessions, some deep-tissue massage, reflexology, or a sauna. However, when all is said and done, the most important thing you can do right now is eat well and rest. Settle down with your broth or juice, read a good book, relax, and let your body clean house.

Old Illnesses Revisited

My mother once told me that deciding to go on a personal pilgrimage was to accept that anything can happen. Detoxing your body is similar in that you can always expect the unexpected to occur. This way you won't be surprised or appalled when what seems like an old illness shows up. As you go deeper into your detox, old health conditions and emotional issues can surface. "Surprise! We never went away. All this time we've been burrowed deep in your body and now we're coming out to play."

Although you might have forgotten the times you were ill or injured in the past, during your detox you could be reminded. This can include emotional issues that were never resolved. When you ask the body to rid itself of toxins, those can be emotional and spiritual toxins as well. What we store in the body will find a way to surface, and a good detoxification can clear out a lot more than the sludge in your large intestine.

If old emotional symptoms come to the surface, just know your body, mind, and soul want to throw them out for good. Rather than suppress the symptom, stay with the program but seek guided counseling to help you resolve and rid it from your life once and for all. Past physical symptoms can come up, but will eventually pass as your body rids itself of poisons accumulated over your lifetime. When you find yourself clearing out the linen closet, just know that's part of the detox as well. Not only will you end up with a clean body, but your house can also be purged of any accumulated waste.

You may want to view your detox program as a pilgrimage of sorts. A journey of the self, for the self. One that brings you full circle, from a healthy child to a sick and toxic adult and back to optimal health again.

Cleansing Layer by Layer

A blending of Eastern and Western modalities has emerged to provide us with a new way of looking at our health and how disease is caused. Integrative, complementary, or alternative medicines are distinct from Western, conventional, or allopathic medicines in that they emerged from Eastern philosophy. They developed from a *holistic view* of the genesis of illness, healing, and body mechanics.

def•i•ni•tion

> A **holistic view** looks at the whole person, including analysis of physical, nutritional, environmental, emotional, social, spiritual, and lifestyle values. It encompasses all stated modalities of diagnosis and treatment, including drugs and surgery if no safe alternative exists. Holistic medicine focuses on education and responsibility for personal efforts to achieve balance and well-being for each individual.

Integrative and complementary refer to the action of combining alternative modalities among themselves, as well as with conventional treatments, for maximum healing effect. Moreover, integrative and complementary describe the relationship between the modalities and the body itself, where the modalities interact with and enhance the natural healing capacity of the human being.

There are certain health conditions that may need medical support in conjunction with a detoxifying diet, to help eliminate toxins trapped on a deeper level. This can happen in the case of heavy-metal poisoning, chemical exposure, or parasite infestation. In holistic wellness centers, you will often find alternative methods of detoxification married to conventional technology that can help you with this need to go deeper. These detoxification processes can also help to alleviate the Herxheimer reactions you might be experiencing with dietary and lifestyle changes.

> **Pure Insights** _____
>
> Alternative indicates a choice among equals. Where one modality is an alternative to another treatment, it suggests that either might be effective. One might be preferable to the other based on certain factors, but the outcomes are likely to be equal. Using alternative modalities does not imply the dismissal or rejection of the value of conventional medicine.
>
> —Rashmi Gulati, M.D.

Chelation Therapy

Chelation therapy is a safe, effective, and relatively inexpensive treatment to remove heavy metals from the blood, and it has been observed to have a positive effect on cardiovascular disease as well. It involves the intravenous infusion of a prescription medicine called ethylene diamine tetra-acetic acid (EDTA), plus vitamins and minerals at therapeutic dosages. EDTA chelation infusions are administered by slow drip, circulating through the bloodstream and treating the entire arterial system by removing undesirable metals from the body. EDTA helps prevent the production of harmful free radicals through elimination. Arterial disease is responsible for strokes, heart attacks, poor circulation, and memory loss.

Vitamin IV Drip

A vitamin IV drip is often recommended by holistic practitioners for malnourished and toxic individuals. In this particular class of patients, physician-directed IVs may be needed to "jump-start" absorption and utilization of nutrients before regular oral nutrition is introduced.

When nutrients are injected intravenously or intramuscularly, they go straight into the bloodstream, where they can be delivered immediately to the tissues or organs that need them. Some of these nutrients are promptly excreted by the kidneys and liver, but the natural intelligence of the body will retain the nutrients it needs to survive.

A classic multivitamin/mineral infusion may contain:

- 10 to 30 grams of vitamin C
- 100 milligrams B-complex
- 1 milligram vitamin B12
- 5 to 10 milligrams folic acid
- 600 to 2000 milligrams magnesium and calcium

Vitamin infusions are considered safe and effective in providing essential nutrients to a depleted system. For your detox purposes, oral supplements will suffice, but for those of you using the five-week detox program to heal from a serious illness, you may want to add this treatment to your protocol.

The Least You Need to Know

- When your body is cleansing faster than it can eliminate toxins, you will experience the "die-off" reaction, which occurs when toxic microbes in your body are starved of the foods that feed them, such as sugar, dairy, and alcohol.

- The severity of these reactions will vary from person to person depending on immune strength, bowel function, and how your organs of detoxification are working.

- With full awareness of your body, you can use visual diagnosis as a tool to see an illness forming or to prevent one from fully manifesting.

- To counter Herxheimer reactions, your body needs fresh vegetable juices, potassium-rich foods, and lots of water to help wash out the toxins.

- What you store in your body will find a way to surface, whether in the form of emotional, spiritual, or physical toxins.

- Certain health conditions may need more than a detoxifying diet to help eliminate toxins trapped on a deeper level.

Part 3

Ladies and Gentlemen, Start Your Organs

Welcome to your five-week detox program. The next five chapters provide you with a week-by-week progression of the dietary changes you will be making. The first week of any dietary program can be a little confusing because it throws you off your regular schedule of finding and preparing food. Now you have to think about cooking for your family and yourself at the same time. Then there is the confusion in the grocery store of trying to find new products, figuring out how much they cost, and deciding whether you will like how they taste. Don't worry, you'll figure it out with the help of this book, and before long what seemed unfamiliar will become a welcome and comfortable part of your life.

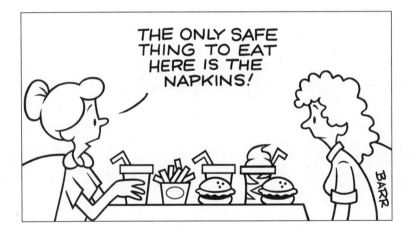

Chapter 9

Week One: Getting Started

In This Chapter

- ◆ Making healthy substitutions for your favorite foods
- ◆ What you can eat
- ◆ Foods to avoid
- ◆ Detox eating guidelines
- ◆ Your week one shopping checklist
- ◆ Meals and snacks for week one

This is the perfect place to begin your detox program. It allows you to transition slowly, avoiding confusion and physical discomfort. Read through the entire chapter first. Get an idea of what you will be eating for this first week. Look over the meals and snacks (and the recipes included in Appendix B) and choose a few that look good to you. Then take the provided shopping list and go shopping. Buy enough food for one week or buy only what the recipes call for. Week two of the detox program (covered in the next chapter) requires a separate food list because you will continue to make dietary changes.

In this chapter, you will find your detox eating guidelines: the foods you can eat, foods you should avoid, a comprehensive shopping list, and meals and snacks using foods you will introduce to your diet. Take it one day at a time and remember: if you follow the guidelines as I have written them, you will get the beneficial results!

One Food at a Time

The sooner you eliminate certain foods, the sooner you begin the detoxification process. For this first week, try to remove one food each day and substitute it with the recommended substitution foods:

> *Eliminate:* All dairy products such as cheese, milk, and yogurt
>
> *Substitute:* Nondairy nut and rice milks, rice cheese, and soy yogurt
>
> *Eliminate:* All wheat products, such as bread, baked goods, soy sauce, and pasta (wheat is in a lot of foods, so read labels carefully)
>
> *Substitute:* Wheat-free pasta, breads, baked goods made with spelt, rice, rye, Kamut, oat, barley, quinoa, millet, amaranth, and buckwheat
>
> *Eliminate:* All refined sugar products and artificial sweeteners, including cookies, cakes, candy, soda pop, diet soda, and ice cream (read labels carefully, sugar and/or artificial sweeteners are hidden in many common products).
>
> *Substitute:* Raw honey, maple syrup, agave syrup, rice syrup, stevia, and xylitol

When human beings evolved from hunter-gatherers to agrarian farmers around 5000 B.C.E., they started by planting grains. Spelt (Triticum spelta) is said to be one of the first grains planted. It is a member of the wheat family but contains more protein, B vitamins, and simple and complex carbohydrates than wheat does. For those unable to tolerate wheat, spelt makes an excellent substitute because it is easier to digest. If you are gluten-intolerant, you should avoid barley, Kamut, rye, spelt, and oats, as well as wheat. Instead, you can eat the nongluten grains, quinoa, millet, amaranth, and brown rice.

Kamut is another high-protein grain that contains 30 percent more protein than wheat. Due to its slightly higher fatty acid content, Kamut can be considered a high-energy grain and compared to wheat, Kamut also contains elevated levels of vitamin E, thiamin, riboflavin, phosphorus, magnesium, zinc, pantothentic acid, copper, and complex carbohydrates. Because of its larger seed size in comparison to wheat, there's less fiber in Kamut than wheat.

Quinoa has it ancient roots in South America, where it has been the staple food for 5,000 years. Known as the "Mother Grain," quinoa has the highest yield of protein than any of the other grains. It is a nongluten grain ideal for people with gluten allergies and diabetics. It is also an alkaline food, whereas other grains are acidic. It is quick and easy to prepare and absolutely delicious.

Amaranth, from the Greek for "never-fading flower," is really an herb, not a grain. It is the seeds that are cooked or ground into a flour and made into bread. Its nutty flavor, high-protein content, and respectable amounts of vitamins and minerals make it a must-have in your diet.

> **Healthy Tidbits**
>
> Amaranth has a sticky texture rather than the fluffy texture of other grains when cooked. When overcooked, it can become gummy. If this happens, all is not lost: just add some dried fruit, nuts, and sweetener, bake it for 20 minutes at 350°F, and a cake is born!

All the substitution foods are readily available in your local natural foods market and/or grocery store. Otherwise, plan ahead and request the store stock the items. You can also order the items online if necessary. See Appendix D for ordering websites.

There's Plenty to Eat

Consider what you usually eat in a week. If you are like most people, you rotate 10 or so different meals over and over again. This is how most people deal with variety in their diet. Now you are faced with changing those 10 recipes and creating new healthy recipes you can live with comfortably. You've been stuck in the 10-meal rut for so long it is hard to imagine what else there is. Use the higher-quality whole foods in your favorite recipes to upgrade rather than eliminate what you love.

Your favorite pasta dish can be made with rice or spelt pasta, organic vegetables, and pasta sauce. Try topping it with soy or rice Parmesan cheese (nondairy). Silken tofu makes a great substitute for ricotta cheese. Place the tofu in the blender with the juice of half a lemon and purée until smooth. Layer in between wheat-free lasagna noodles with tomato sauce and top with grated nondairy mozzarella. Make it for the family without mentioning the substitutions, and they won't notice the difference.

Once you start including the recommended foods into your diet, you will either forget about your favorite 10, or at least only remember them fondly from time to time. You can always have them again after your five weeks are over.

Ideally you should eat five servings of vegetables daily. Try to include greens such as kale, collards, spinach, and curly leaf lettuce. Looking at your dinner plate: 80 percent should be cooked and raw vegetables, with the remaining 20 percent starch or protein. (See Chapter 12 for more on combining foods.)

Eating too many starchy vegetables such as yams, red-skinned potatoes, winter squash, corn on the cob, and lima beans can slow down the detox process, so limit them to three times a week. Remember to make them only 20 percent of your diet.

Fruit is high in sugar and can spike your blood sugar levels when eaten in excess. Limit your fruits to two per day and eat them between meals.

This is a good time to introduce yourself to whole grains. They are easy to prepare, most requiring 2 cups water to 1 cup of grain. Bring to a boil in a saucepan, add a pinch of quality sea salt, cover, reduce heat, and simmer until all the water is absorbed. For maximum digestibility, soak the grain in water while you are at work and cook it when you get home. Sauté some garlic in olive oil and pour over the cooked grain. Mix well and serve as a side dish or toss into a quick vegetable stir-fry and add a can of rinsed black beans.

Cooking times are as follows:

- Millet, amaranth, quinoa, or buckwheat: 20 minutes

- Barley: 30 minutes

- Brown rice: 40 minutes

- Kamut or spelt: 50 minutes

- Whole oats: 90 minutes

Most people know how to throw a few shrimp on the barbie or grill a piece of fish or steak. That doesn't need to change; just make sure the protein is organic and any marinade you use contains recommended ingredients. For animal protein, have fish, shellfish, organic chicken, organic meat, lamb, buffalo, turkey, or organic eggs.

At least one meal a day should be vegetarian. Proteins to use are beans, tofu, tempeh, nuts, seeds, and legumes. Beans are a starch-protein combination, which is why they cause digestive gas to occur. They are easier to digest when presoaked and cooked with a bay leaf, ginger, or a small piece of kombu seaweed. Different cultures have used these foods to reduce the flatulent properties of beans.

> **Pure Insights**
>
> Eating added sugar in various foods and drinks every day is a way of perpetuating chronic over stimulation of the pituitary and pancreas glands. The thyroid and adrenals also feel the brunt of the affront. The false craving and feeling of well-being sugar induces is on a par with the ecstasy experienced when dope takes command in a victim's body.
>
> —Dr. Edward Howell, *Enzyme Nutrition*

Eat nuts and seeds sparingly, and soak or dry roast for easier digestion:

◆ *To soak:* Place a handful of seeds or nuts in a bowl and cover with pure water. Allow to soak overnight in the refrigerator.

◆ *To roast pumpkin, sunflower, and sesame seeds:* Heat a small, heavy skillet over medium-high flame. Add the seeds, reduce heat, and stir the seeds as they roast. When they are lightly browned, remove to a bowl and allow them to cool.

◆ *To roast nuts:* Preheat oven to 350°F. Spread the desired amount of nuts on a baking sheet and bake 10 to 20 minutes, depending on the density of the nut. Cool before using.

Use all the wonderful culinary herbs reviewed in Chapter 6, in both fresh and dry form, when cooking. Feel free to use raw or cooked garlic in your recipes and dressings.

There are four basic types of fat that our bodies need, and they all come from your diet: polyunsaturated, cholesterol, monounsaturated, and saturated fats. Essential for good health are the polyunsaturated omega-3 fatty acids. The best oils to use are the organic cold-pressed oils: extra-virgin olive oil, coconut oil, and ghee (clarified butter).

Olive oil is best unheated to retain the enzymes. Coconut oil is antifungal, antibacterial, and antiviral, and can be used for high-temperature cooking. Ghee is butter with the milk fats removed. This leaves a delicious golden liquid stable at high temperatures. Ghee will contribute a rich buttery taste to your recipes.

Avoid all margarines and have organic butter, but in moderation. You might try having goat's milk butter, which is easier to digest for most people, although the taste may be stronger than cow's butter. It is lovely on a thin slice of steamed whole spelt bread with a smear of raw honey.

There are whole-grain, wheat-free breads and pastas just awaiting your discovery. Use them as you normally would and enjoy the divine taste and texture of these superior flour products. You can keep the breads frozen and remove what you need, then steam or toast. Steaming a dense whole-grain bread softens the texture, as if it just came out of the oven. Place a half inch of water and a steamer basket into a small skillet. Lay the sliced bread on the basket, cover, and allow to steam no more than 10 seconds. Remove immediately.

The sweeteners you can use this week are a mixed bag of high sugars and others that won't cause a spike in your blood sugar:

♦ Rice syrup is a complex sugar, which allows it to be absorbed more slowly. It is not as sweet as you are used to, but it adds a delicate flavor to dessert recipes. One tablespoon of rice syrup has 75 calories, 11 grams of sugar, and 18 grams of carbohydrates.

♦ Agave syrup comes from the agave cactus plant, which is also used to make tequila. It tastes like a cross between maple and rice syrup and is safe for diabetics. One tablespoon of agave syrup has 60 calories, 16 grams of sugar, and 16 grams of carbohydrates.

♦ Raw honey is a high-sugar food with traces of B vitamins. One tablespoon of honey has 64 calories, 17 grams of carbohydrates, and 17 grams of sugar.

♦ Maple syrup is a concentrated sugar tapped from the maple tree. It takes 40 gallons of maple sap for 1 gallon of syrup. It has fewer calories than honey at 52 calories per tablespoon, 13 grams of carbohydrate, and 12 grams of sugar. Plus, it contains high amounts of the minerals manganese and zinc.

def•i•ni•tion

Miso is a fermented paste loaded with enzymes, with a salty taste. It is made from soy, barley, rice, or beans. The darker the miso, the longer the aging process. For a light flavor, try the mellow white miso. For winter soups, use the dark barley or rice miso.

Drink half your weight in ounces of spring, distilled, or filtered water daily. Also use it for all your cooking. Organic herbal teas like dandelion root, burdock root, peppermint, and chamomile are an excellent addition to your diet.

When salting your foods, use a high-quality mineral-rich sea salt or tamari, the wheat-free alternative to regular soy sauce. For added flavor, sprinkle some in your stir-fries. You can also add *miso* to soups, salad dressings, sauces, and marinades.

Use natural, organic raw and roasted nut and seed butters in moderation. Almond butter is the perfect replacement for peanut butter. Sesame seed butter (tahini) can be blended with water, vinegar, white miso, green onions, garlic, and lemon juice as a salad dressing or topping for your grains.

What to Avoid

The foods you want to avoid are the classic bad guys of the refined, junk-food world. You've read all about them, and know they are the root of all your ills. Say good-bye and good riddance.

Avoid all refined and processed foods of any kind, such as cookies, cakes, luncheon meats, soy powder, white bread, frozen dinners, and fast foods.

Also avoid all refined and processed sugars, including fructose, cane crystals, and corn syrup; diet products with artificial sweeteners such as aspartame (NutraSweet), sucralose (Splenda), and saccharin (Sweet & Low); all dairy products except organic butter; regular and decaffeinated coffee (except in week one to ease off of regular coffee); and peanut butter, because it may contain the aflatoxin mold.

Some people may want to immediately give up everything in one day, but take heed. I strongly suggest you go slowly so as not to detoxify too quickly. Remember, for every food you remove from your diet, make sure you have something to replace it with. This way you won't be tempted to return to the foods you just eliminated.

The classic scenario is you get through the first week doing everything perfectly and decide to go out to dinner with friends.

> **Detox Alert**
>
> The aflatoxin mold is found in corn and peanuts. It comes from the aspergillus flavus, one of a type of mold considered to be a carcinogen. Aflatoxin is considered a cancer-causing substance in humans and animals by both the FDA and world health authorities.

Feeling pretty sure of yourself, you refuse the bread and butter, but you're really hungry and love the bread they serve. Remind yourself that you can always come back and have that slice of bread in five weeks, when you've finished the detox program, or bring along some spelt crackers to eat instead.

Don't Stuff Your Belly

Stuffing your belly is a major cause of indigestion and weight gain. Your stomach is about the size of your hand, and though it can stretch, your stomach needs room to break down the food you've eaten, mix it with gastric juices, and send it on to your small intestine. Eat until you are almost full, leaving plenty of room for digestion.

> **Healthy Tidbits**
>
> For optimal digestion, try to complete eating no later than 7:30 P.M.

Your teeth are the first step in the process of digestion. Be sure to grind food to liquid before swallowing. It is important to eat slowly and chew each bite completely. This allows the salivary glands to release essential digestive enzymes. You can accomplish about one third of your digestion in your mouth if you chew each bite 30 to 40 times.

Your stomach was not designed to break down huge chunks of animal fiber, large bites of pizza, or whole nuts. Chewing slowly and not overeating ensures that your body is able to absorb the highest amount of nutrients from each meal. Many digestive problems can clear up simply by chewing your food.

Before You Begin ...

Before each week begins, look over the "Meals and Snacks" section for that week to see what foods you'll need. A shopping checklist of these items is ready for you to take along to your local foods market (make a copy of the list to take with you). Remember to buy organically grown foods whenever possible, as discussed in Chapter 5. Once you have that week's food items in your cupboard, you can move easily from day to day without interrupting the detoxification process.

Feel free to improvise with your own recipes, based on the "There's Plenty to Eat" section earlier in this chapter.

Week One Shopping Checklist

FRUITS:

❑ Lemons

❑ Blueberries (fresh and frozen)

❑ Apples

❑ Bananas

❑ Red grapes

❑ Strawberries

❑ Pears

❑ Kiwis

❑ Pomegranates

❑ Peaches (frozen)

❑ Raisins

❑ Dried cranberries (sweetened with fruit juice)

VEGETABLES:

❑ Spinach

❑ Arugula

❑ Watercress

❑ Mesclun salad mix

❑ Lettuce

❑ Bok choy

❑ Carrots

❑ Celery

❑ Red onions

❑ Green onions

❑ Sweet onions

❑ Garlic

❑ Kale

❑ Fennel bulbs

❑ Broccoli

❑ Broccoli rabe

❑ Green beans

❑ Asparagus

❑ Tomatoes

❑ Zucchini

❑ Baby bella mushrooms

❑ Red peppers

❑ Jalapeño peppers

❑ Avocadoes

BEVERAGES:

❑ Decaffeinated coffee (for making the transition)

❑ Soy/rice milk

❑ Cranberry juice (unsweetened)

❑ Apple juice

❑ Tomato juice

❑ Distilled or filtered water

❑ Sleepytime tea (made by Celestial Seasonings)

❑ Dandelion tea

❑ Camomile tea

❑ Rooibos tea

❑ Coconut milk

SWEETENERS:

❑ Raw honey

❑ Stevia

❑ Maple syrup

OILS AND CONDIMENTS:

❑ Extra-virgin olive oil

❑ Coconut oil

❑ Balsamic vinegar

❑ Vegenaise (vegan mayonnaise)

❑ Apple cider vinegar

❑ White miso

❑ Sea salt

❑ Salsa

NUTS AND SEEDS:

☐ Almonds

☐ Walnuts

☐ Pumpkin seeds

☐ Pecans

☐ Almond butter

☐ Flax meal

☐ Fiber powder

HERBS AND SPICES:

☐ Fresh basil

☐ Fresh parsley

☐ Ginger root

☐ Cayenne pepper

☐ Cinnamon

PROTEIN:

☐ Wild salmon

☐ Sea scallops

☐ Shrimp

☐ Turkey burgers

☐ Turkey sausage

☐ Chicken breasts

☐ Steak

☐ Lamb chops

☐ Hemp protein powder

☐ Firm tofu

☐ Eggs

GRAINS:

☐ Cream of rice cereal

☐ Buckwheat pancake mix

☐ Steel-cut oatmeal

☐ Wheat-free waffles

☐ Wheat-free hamburger buns

☐ Spelt crackers

☐ Spelt tortillas

☐ Spelt bread

☐ Wild rice

☐ Short-grain brown rice

☐ Spelt angel hair pasta

☐ Brown rice pasta

EXTRAS:

☐ Soy yogurt

☐ Organic butter

☐ Probiotics

☐ Wooden shish kabob skewers

Week One Meals and Snacks

Week one menu items are designed to be quick and easy to keep up with your life-style. They also work for those of you not comfortable in the kitchen. Don't be afraid to substitute an ingredient you prefer, as long as it is on the preceding detox foods list. Begin each morning with the juice of half a lemon in water to prepare your digestive system and soften the liver. Sweeten with honey, or look ahead to Chapter 10 and read all about using the herb stevia as a sweetener. Most of all, enjoy the adventure of exploring new tastes, new foods, and the physical feelings of well-being that these foods bring to your body.

Day One

Upon rising: The juice of ½ lemon in 8 oz. water, sweetened with honey.

Breakfast: Buckwheat pancakes with organic blueberries and maple syrup; tea or decaffeinated coffee with nondairy milk.

Snack: Spelt crackers or an apple with almond butter.

Lunch: Turkey burger on wheat-free bun with lettuce, tomato, onion, 1 tsp. Vegenaise mixed with 2 tsp. salsa; arugula mesclun salad with balsamic vinegar and olive oil dressing.

Snack: Fresh blueberries or handful of toasted almonds.

Dinner: Broiled or grilled salmon; spelt angel-hair pasta tossed with garlic sautéed in olive oil; steamed broccoli topped with toasted walnuts.

Before bedtime: The juice of ½ lemon in 8 oz. water, sweetened with honey. Take your probiotics.

Day Two

Upon rising: The juice of ½ lemon in 8 oz. water, sweetened with honey.

Breakfast: Veggie omelet with spelt toast and butter; rooibos tea with rice milk and honey.

Snack: Toasted pumpkin seeds with raisins.

Lunch: Mixed-green salad with baked tofu or grilled chicken; vegetable soup; spelt bread with almond butter.

Snack: Banana Apple Smoothie: purée in blender 1 frozen banana; half an organic apple, chopped; 1 cup apple juice or water; ½ tsp. cinnamon, and 1 TB. hemp protein powder. Sweeten to taste.

Dinner: Broccoli rabe and turkey sausage; wild rice topped with toasted almonds; fresh green salad.

Before bedtime: The juice of ½ lemon in 8 oz. water, sweetened with honey. Take your probiotics.

Day Three

Upon rising: The juice of ½ lemon in 8 oz. water, sweetened with honey.

Breakfast: Blueberry Fruit Smoothie: purée in a blender 8 oz. water, 1 TB. hemp protein powder, 1 TB. flax meal, 1 tsp. fiber powder, and ½ cup frozen blueberries; sweeten to taste.

Snack: Tofu Nut Butter (see recipe in Appendix B) on spelt crackers.

Lunch: Roasted vegetables and sliced, grilled chicken rolled up in a spelt tortilla with Vegenaise; fresh green salad.

Snack: Coconut Ginger Smoothie: purée in blender ¼ cup apple juice; ¼ cup unsweetened coconut milk; ½ banana; ¼ tsp. fresh ginger root, peeled; and ½ cup crushed ice or 2 small ice cubes. Sweeten to taste.

Dinner: Grilled Chicken with Pesto (see recipe in Appendix B); pan-grilled asparagus; water-cooked kale; green salad with lemon–olive oil vinaigrette.

Before bedtime: Unsweetened cranberry juice and water, sweetened with honey. Take your probiotics.

Day Four

Upon rising: The juice of ½ lemon in 8 oz. water, sweetened with honey.

Breakfast: Bowl of steel-cut oatmeal topped with fresh blueberries.

Snack: Sliced kiwis.

Lunch: Watercress Mesclun Salad (see recipe in Appendix B).

Snack: Spicy Vegetable Smoothie: purée in blender 1 cup organic tomato juice; ¼ avocado; ½ tsp. jalapeño pepper, chopped; ¼ tsp. dried cayenne pepper; ¼ cup chopped onion; ¼ cup chopped parsley; and 2 cloves garlic, peeled.

Dinner: Grilled salmon, green beans sautéed with onions and garlic; fresh spinach salad.

Before bedtime: Unsweetened cranberry juice and water, sweetened with honey. Take your probiotics.

Day Five

Upon rising: The juice of ½ lemon in 8 oz. water, sweetened with honey.

Breakfast: Wheat-free waffles with fresh blueberries and maple syrup.

Snack: Fresh pear with unsweetened soy yogurt, topped with cinnamon and drizzled with maple syrup.

Lunch: Grilled chicken on spelt bread, with lettuce, tomato, and Vegenaise; fresh spinach salad.

Snack: Raisins; fruit juice–sweetened cranberries; walnuts.

Dinner: Garlic sautéed shrimp; wheat-free rice pasta and fresh tomato sauce; steamed vegetable medley; mesclun salad with lemon-garlic dressing.

Before bedtime: Cup of dandelion tea. Take your probiotics.

Day Six

Upon rising: The juice of ½ lemon in 8 oz. water, sweetened with honey.

Breakfast: Poached eggs with cooked spinach; wheat-free toast and butter.

Snack: Sliced strawberries with unsweetened soy yogurt, drizzled with maple syrup.

Lunch: Sliced steak or chicken with avocado; arugula; watercress salad and lemon–olive oil dressing.

Snack: Cooked brown rice mixed with diced carrot, celery, and red onion; tossed with olive oil and lemon juice or apple cider vinegar.

Dinner: Rosemary Balsamic Chicken Kabobs; Watercress Pomegranate Salad (see recipes in Appendix B).

Before bedtime: Cup of chamomile tea. Take your probiotics.

Day Seven

Upon rising: The juice of ½ lemon in 8 oz. water, sweetened with honey.

Breakfast: Cream of rice cereal with maple syrup and fresh blueberries.

Snack: Handful of grapes.

Lunch: Grilled lamb chops; Kale Walnut Salad (see recipe in Appendix B).

Snack: Peachy Smoothie: purée in blender 1 cup frozen peach slices; ½ banana, sliced; 3 TB. unsweetened soy yogurt; ¼ cup apple juice; and ½ cup rice milk. Sweeten to taste.

Dinner: Grilled scallops; cooked brown rice tossed with sautéed garlic; grilled asparagus; fresh green salad.

Before bedtime: The juice of ½ lemon in 8 oz. water, sweetened with honey. Take your probiotics.

The Least You Need to Know

- Eliminate dairy, refined sugar, and wheat products.
- Adapt the substitute foods to your recipes.
- Eat five servings of vegetables each day.
- Soak or roast nuts and seeds before eating.
- Eat only wheat-free breads and pasta.
- Read the labels for nondairy milks to avoid added sugar.

Chapter 10

Week Two: Going Deeper

In This Chapter

- Continuing food elimination
- Getting rid of flour
- Benefits of nongluten grains
- New foods to enjoy
- Your week two shopping checklist
- Meals and snacks for week two

If you managed to eliminate dairy, wheat, and sugar from your diet, congratulations! For most of you, week one was a major transition, and now you can reap the rewards. Week two continues to ease you away from foods that can stress your body. This will allow you to detox on a deeper level. Make sure you eat enough of the recommended foods. This is not a low-calorie, low-fat diet. It is a balance of protein, carbohydrates, and fats. These can be spread out over three meals and two snacks, or five small meals every two hours. You know best how you like to eat, so go to it.

In this chapter, you will find instructions for moving to the next level in your detox. Dry goods and sweeteners you bought for week one and did not use completely can be put aside for now; you will come back to them later. Leftover bread can be frozen, as can any flour and nuts. Chapter 13 will show you how these new sweeteners, breads, and flours can be added to your diet to help keep you healthy for a lifetime.

Foods to Eliminate

There are a few more foods for you to eliminate in week two. Some, like bread and sweeteners, you eat every day and you may feel lost without them. Just remember that once your detox is over, you can return them to your diet.

For this week, try to remove one food each day and substitute the recommended foods:

Eliminate: All flour products: pasta, bread, baked goods, dry cereals, and chips.

Substitute: Nongluten whole grains like quinoa, brown rice, amaranth, and millet. This includes any bread or pasta made from spelt or rice flour. These next few weeks call for eating the whole grain before it is processed to flour.

Eliminate: All forms of sugar.

Substitute: Stevia and xylitol.

Eliminate: Wine, beer, and all forms of alcohol.

Substitute: Fresh vegetable juices, herbal tea, pure water, and homemade nut and seed milks.

Eliminate: Regular and decaffeinated coffees and teas.

Substitute: Fresh lemon and water, herbal teas, grain coffee, and unsweetened cranberry juice.

Eliminate: Pasteurized fruit juice.

Substitute: Fresh organic fruit and vegetable juice. Try having one glass a day.

def•i•ni•tion

Excitotoxins are food additives that destroy nerve cells in the brain. Common excitotoxins found in the diet are MSG, aspartame, and hydrolyzed vegetable protein.

Eliminate: Foods containing MSG and hydrolyzed vegetable protein. These are *excitotoxins* and are in the same toxic category as aspartame. Read labels carefully, as MSG is present in almost all processed foods. It can even be in foods labeled "No MSG."

Eliminate: Unfermented soy products. Soybeans have one of the highest glutamate levels of any plant food.

When soy is hydrolyzed, glutamate is released and the soy protein isolates. Glutamate levels in soy are higher than products containing MSG. Unfermented soy products contain a mixture of toxins that can destroy the nervous system.

Substitute: Tempeh and miso; tofu (in moderation).

> **Detox Alert**
>
> You get very high glutamate levels in the blood after eating a meal containing MSG. You're stimulating all of the glutamate receptors. That's why some people get explosive diarrhea, because it stimulates the receptors in the esophagus and small bowel. Others may develop irritable bowel, or if they have irritable bowel, it makes it a lot worse. If they have reflux, it makes that a lot worse.
>
> —Dr. Russell Blaylock, author of *Excitotoxins, The Taste That Kills*

Eliminate: All foods containing hydrogenated or partially hydrogenated oils or trans-fatty acids.

Substitute: Cold-pressed organic oils. Trans fatty acids raise LDL (bad) cholesterol and lower HDL (good) cholesterol, increasing the chance of heart disease, stroke, and diabetes.

Eliminate: All nuts and nut butters, both raw and roasted.

Substitute: Sunflower, pumpkin, and sesame seeds; also pine nuts, which are really seeds.

Eliminate: Commercial iodized salt.

Substitute: Mineral-rich sea salt, tamari soy sauce, miso, herbs, and sea-vegetable condiments.

> **Pure Insights**
>
> Table salt should be dropped from the diet. We do not need it when we have plenty of greens every day. To change from it, use vegetized salt purchased in your health food store. Vegetable concentrates in powdered form and herbs are also excellent seasonings.
>
> —Bernard Jensen, Ph.D.

Nongluten Grains

There are two categories of grain: gluten grains such as barley, oats, rye, wheat, buckwheat, spelt, and Kamut; and nongluten grains like quinoa, rice, millet, and amaranth.

Gluten is what makes the dough stretch and stick together when making bread, cakes, or pizza dough. Nongluten grains do not have that same elasticity. Gluten is the protein in grains and can be very difficult to digest. A weak digestive system overloaded with gluten grains can result in the following health conditions:

- ◆ Chronic indigestion
- ◆ Gas and bloating
- ◆ Celiac disease
- ◆ Allergies
- ◆ Candida albicans
- ◆ Mental illness
- ◆ Multiple sclerosis

Our ancestors consumed a diet high in whole grains, but they made sure to soak them 7 to 24 hours before cooking. This process ensures that the phytic acids present in all grains are neutralized. Phytic acid binds up minerals and makes them impossible to absorb. Soaking eliminates phytic acid, allowing for a more complete absorption of these nutrients. Soaking and cooking grains properly may take a bit more time and consideration, but it will provide a healthier and more digestible food.

Eliminating gluten grains in week two helps ease digestive stress. Because most people are not aware they have a gluten intolerance, it will be good to take a few weeks away from these grains to find out.

Flour Products

Flour is ground and processed grains. Once the grain has been broken and exposed to the air, its volatile oils begin to go rancid if not used within a short time. Flour combined with water, salt, and heat can begin to act like glue in your intestines. This creates a hard, flour-based impaction and can lead to constipation and bloating.

Healthy Tidbits

When storing flour for long periods of time, keep it in the freezer to ensure it stays fresh.

Eating whole grains, on the other hand, acts as a natural intestinal broom that helps to break down impacted feces and eliminate them slowly over time.

You can substitute mochi, a Japanese product made from pounded sweet rice, for bread these next few weeks. Traditionally it is used for stamina and as a blood strengthener. Mochi comes in a block you can cut into squares and bake. I prefer to slice it long and thin, and place in a heated waffle iron. Cook as you would a waffle and top with butter. Mochi comes as cinnamon/raisin, sesame/garlic, cashew/date, plain, and pizza-flavored. All are delicious and easy to prepare.

Introduce New Foods

"Letting go of the familiar to experience the unknown" is what is called for when changing to a whole-foods diet. See if you can introduce a new fruit, vegetable, grain, or protein each day. The green leafy vegetable family is a good place to begin. Plan your meals to be made up of 80 percent cooked and raw vegetables and 20 percent starch and/or protein.

Dark Leafy Greens

Eating dark-green leafy vegetables is one of the best things you can do for your daily diet. They are an excellent source of vitamin A, vitamin C, and calcium. You can replace dairy products with these calcium-rich vegetables, along with the sea vegetables kelp, dulse, nori, arame, and hijiki. They are also great sources of fiber.

The darker leaves have even more of these important nutrients. Consider some of the others from this same nutritious plant family:

- *Collard greens* have an earthy flavor and are rich in vitamin A and calcium. They are best when boiled briefly, cooled, chopped, then added to soups or stir-fries.

- *Arugula* has a distinctive, almost peppery taste. Rich in vitamins A and C and calcium, it is best eaten raw in salads.

- *Dandelion greens* have a slightly bitter flavor and are rich in vitamin A and calcium. Young spring dandelion greens can be eaten raw in salads. Older greens can be lightly boiled until just tender, cooled, chopped, and sautéed with garlic in olive oil.

- *Kale* has a slightly bitter cabbagelike flavor and is rich in vitamins A and C, calcium, folic acid, and potassium. Eating raw kale may cause digestive upset for some people. Kale is best eaten in soups, as a cooked salad, or sautéed with olive oil and garlic and spread on a pizza.

- *Mustard greens* have a hot, spicy flavor, and are rich in vitamins A and C and calcium. Mustard greens can be prepared the same way as dandelion greens. They can also be eaten raw in salads, or in stir-fries and soups.

- *Spinach* has a sweet flavor, and is rich in vitamins A and C, iron, and calcium. It is best eaten raw in salads, layered in pasta dishes, or lightly steamed.

- *Swiss chard* has a taste similar to spinach. It is rich in vitamins K and C and calcium. Swiss chard can be eaten raw in salads, or lightly sautéed with garlic and olive oil.

- *Chicory* has a slightly bitter flavor, and is rich in vitamins K and C and calcium. Chicory is best eaten with other greens in salad, or in soups and pasta sauces.

As you can see, most green vegetables are eaten raw in salads, or mixed with lettuce, to help modify a bitter taste. To cook dark-green leafy vegetables, you can add them to a soup, steam, or water-cook them. Once cooked, cut the leaves into smaller pieces and add them to garlic sautéed in oil. Have as a side dish to protein and vegetables for a complete meal!

To water-cook the greens, pour ½ inch of water in a skillet, add the washed and stemmed greens, cover and cook over medium heat until just tender, then run under cool water, drain, and chop. Always keep some on hand to use in a quick sauté with sliced garlic and olive oil.

Stevia

Stevia rebaudiana is an herb originally grown in Paraguay and Brazil. It is the glycosides and steviosides in the leaves that make it extremely sweet and yet virtually calorie-free. It has been used as a prepackaged replacement for sugar and artificial sweeteners in many countries. It is safe for diabetics, hypoglycemics, and those with Candida albicans.

Healthy Tidbits _____

Research conducted by Purdue University's Dental Science Research Group reported that consuming stevia may actually help prevent cavities.

The unprocessed stevia leaves, when ground to a powder, are 15 times sweeter than table sugar. Refined stevia can be 300 times sweeter. Stevia provides a delicious, safe alternative to the dangers of refined sugar and artificial sweeteners.

When baking with stevia, 1 teaspoon of refined stevia powder is equivalent to 1 cup of sugar. Stevia has a slight licorice aftertaste that is not unpleasant. In my baking I like to use half a teaspoon of refined stevia powder with half a cup of xylitol. This gives me the sweetness I want and the stevia aftertaste is disguised by the xylitol, which provides body to the recipe.

Xylitol

Four to twelve grams of xylitol a day can help reduce dental cavities. Use it to sweeten tea and desserts. It is also sold in mints and gum. Most xylitol today is made from corn, but it is best when derived from birch bark trees, which are not harmed in the harvesting process. Xylitol is perfect for baking, dissolves quickly, and looks and tastes like sugar but has no aftertaste or side effects. Xylitol …

- ◆ Contains half the calories of sugar.
- ◆ Does not promote tooth decay and gum disease.
- ◆ Is metabolized very slowly, which prevents sugar "highs" and "lows."
- ◆ Is safe to use if you have diabetes, hypoglycemia, chronic fatigue syndrome, Candida albicans, or any condition caused by sugar imbalance.

Actually, xylitol is found naturally in fruits, berries, mushrooms, lettuce, hardwood, and corncobs. Include it slowly into your diet, because it can cause some digestive rumbling when taken in excess.

Week Two Shopping Checklist

FRUITS:

❑ Lemons

❑ Limes

❑ Peaches

❑ Granny Smith apples

❑ Strawberries

❑ Pineapple

❑ Kiwis

❑ Blueberries

❑ Pears

❑ Raisins

VEGETABLES:

❑ Spinach (fresh or frozen)

❑ Baby spinach

❑ Arugula

❑ Watercress

❑ Mesclun salad mix

❑ Red leaf lettuce

❑ Kale

❑ Escarole

❑ Asparagus

❑ Broccoli rabe

❑ Carrots

❏ Celery

❏ Beets

❏ Fennel bulbs

❏ Onions

❏ Red onions

❏ Green onions

❏ Garlic

❏ Green beans

❏ Spaghetti squash

❏ Snow peas

❏ Sweet potatoes

❏ Cabbage

❏ Cucumbers

❏ Wild mushrooms

❏ Tomatoes

❏ Zucchini

❏ Red peppers

LIQUIDS AND BEVERAGES:

❏ Chamomile tea

❏ Dandelion tea

❏ Rice milk

❏ Distilled or filtered water

❏ Tomato juice

❏ Coconut milk

❏ Cranberry juice (unsweetened)

❏ Vegetable stock

SWEETENERS:

❏ Stevia

❏ Xylitol

OILS AND CONDIMENTS:

❏ Apple cider vinegar

❏ Extra-virgin olive oil

❏ White miso

❏ Flax meal

❏ Flaxseed oil

❏ Fiber powder

❏ Sesame oil

❏ Rice vinegar

❏ Sea salt

❏ Umeboshi vinegar

❏ Butter

SEEDS:

❏ Sunflower

❏ Pumpkin

❏ Tahini (sesame butter)

HERBS AND SPICES:

❏ Parsley

❏ Ginger

❏ Cayenne pepper

❏ Dill

❏ Basil

❏ Cinnamon

❏ Curry

❏ Cumin

❏ Turmeric

PROTEIN:

❑ Wild salmon

❑ Tilapia

❑ Halibut

❑ Chicken

❑ Lamb

❑ Extra-firm tofu

❑ Eggs

GRAINS:

❑ Cream of rice cereal

❑ Quinoa

❑ Short-grain brown rice

❑ Millet

❑ Mochi (plain and cinnamon raisin)

BEANS:

❑ Cannellini

❑ Lentils

❑ Chickpeas

PREPARED FOOD:

❑ Vegetarian chili

❑ Dolmades (stuffed grape leaves)

❑ Hummus

❑ Marinara sauce (no added sweeteners)

Week Two Meals and Snacks

As you let go of flour, sugar, caffeine, alcohol, and pasteurized fruit juice this week, make sure you have alternate foods to replace them. This week, include a fiber drink in the morning and begin to sweeten your lemon water and tea with stevia or xylitol. There are still plenty of foods to choose from, as you will see from the next seven-day menu plan.

Day One

Upon rising: The juice of ½ lemon in 8 oz. water, sweetened with stevia; fiber powder or 1 TB. flax meal in water (can also be added to a fruit smoothie).

Breakfast: Cream of rice cereal; fresh strawberries; 1 TB. sunflower seeds.

Snack: One Granny Smith apple.

Lunch: Brown rice; cooked kale; beans or chicken; fresh green salad with apple cider vinegar, garlic, and extra-virgin olive oil.

Snack: Toasted pumpkin seeds; raisins.

Dinner: Grilled lamb; asparagus; garlic-sautéed broccoli rabe; salad greens; grated carrots and beets with Tahini Lemon Dressing (see recipe in Appendix B).

Before bedtime: The juice of ½ lemon in 8 oz. water, sweetened with stevia. Take your probiotics.

Day Two

Upon rising: The juice of ½ lemon in 8 oz. water, sweetened with stevia; fiber powder or 1 TB. flax meal in water.

Breakfast: Organic eggs; cooked spinach; plain mochi.

Snack: Fresh vegetable juice: in a juice extractor, process until smooth 2 carrots, 3-inch piece ginger, and 1 apple.

Lunch: Arugula, mesclun, and watercress salad with wild salmon.

Snack: Pineapple Coconut Smoothie: purée in blender 1 cup fresh pineapple, ¼ cup unsweetened coconut milk, and 1 cup rice milk. Sweeten with stevia to taste.

Dinner: Steamed spaghetti squash with marinara sauce and cannellini beans; fresh green salad with fennel, red onion, and garlic lemon dressing.

Before bedtime: Cup of dandelion tea. Take your probiotics.

Day Three

Upon rising: The juice of ½ lemon in 8 oz. water, sweetened with stevia; fiber powder or 1 TB. flax meal in water.

Breakfast: Apple Strawberry Smoothie: purée in blender ½ green apple, 8 strawberries, and scoop of fiber powder; sweeten to taste with stevia.

Snack: One hard-boiled egg; tomato juice.

Lunch: Baked tilapia; green beans; quinoa tossed with sautéed garlic; fresh mesclun salad.

Dinner: Vegetarian chili over brown rice; fresh spinach salad.

Before bedtime: The juice of ½ lemon in 8 oz. water, sweetened with stevia. Take your probiotics.

Day Four

Upon rising: The juice of ½ lemon in 8 oz. water, sweetened with stevia; fiber powder or 1 TB. flax powder in water.

Breakfast: Soft Brown Rice and Quinoa (see recipe in Appendix B).

Snack: One ripe peach.

Lunch: Spinach and salmon salad (toss together green onions, baby spinach, cooked snow peas, sesame oil, rice vinegar, Umeboshi vinegar, and lime juice; top with grilled salmon).

Snack: Fresh vegetable juice: in a juice extractor, process until smooth 2 carrots, ¼ beet, 2 stalks celery, and a handful of parsley.

Dinner: Hummus platter with grilled vegetables; dolmades (stuffed grape leaves); green salad.

Before bedtime: Cup of chamomile tea. Take your probiotics.

Day Five

Upon rising: The juice of ½ lemon in 8 oz. water, sweetened with stevia; fiber powder or 1 TB. flax meal in water.

Breakfast: Eggs Florentine (see recipe in Appendix B).

Snack: Two kiwis.

Lunch: Chicken Garlic Soup (see recipe in Appendix B); cooked millet; fresh green salad.

Snack: Fresh vegetable juice: in a juice extractor, process until smooth 2 carrots, 3 celery stalks, small wedge of cabbage, and ½ cucumber.

Dinner: Risotto with Wild Mushrooms (see recipe in Appendix B).

Before bedtime: The juice of ½ lemon in 8 oz. water, sweetened with stevia. Take your probiotics.

Day Six

Upon rising: The juice of ½ lemon in 8 oz. water, sweetened with stevia; fiber powder or 1 TB. flax meal in water.

Breakfast: Vegetable omelet; cinnamon raisin mochi.

Snack: One Granny Smith apple.

Lunch: Roasted Salmon with Lemon Garlic Sauce (see recipes in Appendix B).

Snack: Fresh vegetable juice: in a juice extractor, process until smooth 2 carrots, 3 stalks celery, 2 tomatoes, 4 spinach leaves, and 4 kale leaves. Pour juice into a blender and add 3 sprigs dill, juice of 1 lemon, 1 clove garlic, ½ tsp. cayenne pepper, and 1 tsp. Umeboshi vinegar. Purée until smooth.

Dinner: Quinoa Lettuce Wraps (see recipe in Appendix B); lentil vegetable soup.

Before bedtime: Cup of dandelion tea. Take your probiotics.

Day Seven

Upon rising: The juice of ½ lemon in 8 oz. water, sweetened with stevia; fiber powder or 1 TB. flax meal in water.

Breakfast: Mochi waffles with cinnamon/stevia sprinkle (in a shaker container combine 4 parts cinnamon to 1 part stevia powder and mix well); butter; fresh blueberries.

Snack: One pear.

Lunch: Stir-fried vegetables; baked halibut; fresh green salad.

Snack: Fresh vegetable juice: in a juice extractor, process until smooth ½ cucumber, 2 stalks celery, 2 kale leaves with stems, and 2 carrots.

Dinner: Vegetable Shish Kabobs (see recipe in Appendix B); watercress and spinach salad.

Before bedtime: The juice of ½ lemon in 8 oz. water, sweetened with stevia. Take your probiotics.

The Least You Need to Know

♦ During week two, eliminate all flour products, including nonwheat breads, pastas, and baked goods.

♦ Eliminate all sweeteners but stevia and xylitol during week two.

♦ Make leafy green vegetables such as kale, spinach, swiss chard, collards, broccoli rabe, and dandelion greens a regular staple in your diet.

♦ Mochi can be an excellent substitute for bread when sliced thinly and cooked in a waffle iron.

♦ Avoid all foods containing the family of excitotoxins: aspartame, MSG, and hydrolyzed vegetable protein.

♦ Feel free to create your own recipes using the bounty of delicious fruits, vegetables, whole grains, proteins, and teas available for you in week two.

Week Three: Time to Fast

In This Chapter

The third week of your detox introduces you to the age-old practice of fasting. This can be challenging for those unused to going without solid food for 24 hours. You may have fasted during religious holidays and remember feeling hungry, tired, cranky, and glad when it was over. After two weeks without refined sugar, caffeine, and junk food, you should be ready to take this next week to move into a day or two of fasting and return to eating whole foods.

In this chapter, you will find descriptions for four different fasting programs, with instructions and recipes. Read through each one and choose the program that appeals to you. Listen to how your body responds to what you are reading. Let your body tell you. If you are unsure, I outline how to choose the program that's right for you.

About Fasting

Fasting is intentionally going without solid food for one or more days. Fasting is not a starvation diet. Its purpose can be religious, spiritual, health-related, or for weight loss. It is one of the most overlooked and yet most beneficial health practices you can experience. It is effective, safe, humbling, enlightening, frustrating, and remarkable. You are literally giving your body a rest from having to digest food 24 hours a day.

Let's say you buy a new car and drive it home, but instead of turning off the engine you leave it running all night, then drive to work in the morning. Again, instead of turning off the engine you leave it running in the parking lot all day and drive it home at night and, yes, leave it running overnight. Imagine doing this day in and day out, never turning it off, pouring gas in the tank to keep it going. After a while the engine will overheat, run out of oil, and break down.

This is similar to how the body is treated. In the morning you gas it up with stimulants and food, eat on and off throughout the day, and have a snack before bedtime. The next day you start eating all over again. Basically, you never stop putting food in your mouth and your digestive system has no chance to rest and detoxify properly.

Pure Insights

There have been some very well done studies on fasting that are entirely scientifically credible. For example, fasting has been shown to be effective in treating high blood pressure, however, medical journals won't publish the research.

—T. Colin Campbell, Ph.D., professor of nutrition and biochemistry at Cornell University

The benefits of fasting can easily counterbalance that strain:

- Fasting rejuvenates the body to a cellular level.
- Fasting is an excellent anti-aging practice.
- Fasting rids the body of toxins, chemicals, and sludge.
- Fasting energizes the whole body.
- Fasting can help eliminate addictions.
- Fasting can improve your sex life.
- Fasting requires little time for food preparation.
- Fasting calms and focuses your mind.
- Fasting is a safe and effective way to detoxify.
- Fasting has been safely practiced for centuries.

You burn a lot of calories just digesting food, but with your digestive system at rest you should have extra energy. You may not even need as much sleep as usual. Make it to 3 P.M. without eating, and the day is almost over. This will help you make it to bedtime. While fasting, many people find themselves doing light cleaning and organizing around the house. Your internal cleansing spills over to your external environment as well.

Choosing Your Fast

When deciding which fast is right for you, consider the diet you followed before beginning the detox program. If you regularly ate the Standard American Diet (see Chapter 3), excessive in acid-forming foods—meat, chicken, fish, salt, flour products, oils, drugs, and legumes—the Fresh-Juice Fast or Master Cleanse would be a good counterbalance. If much of your diet consisted of raw fruits and salads, sugar, dairy, and alcohol, the Mono-Food Fast would be a good counterbalance.

If you must continue taking prescription medications, the Mono-Food Fast or the Raw-Food Fast in this chapter, or the Brown Rice Fast in Chapter 14, would work for you.

Healthy Tidbits

During fasting days, eliminate digestive enzymes, probiotics, and supplements.

Helping Things Along

There are a few things you can do to assist your body to eliminate toxins:

- Take a sauna or steam bath before or after the fasting period. In this way you can receive the detoxing benefits without feeling light-headed and dizzy when combining fasting with high heat.

- Take a shower and alternate between hot water for one minute, then switch to cold water for one minute. Repeat this process several times, going only as hot or cold as your body will allow. This helps to stimulate the body and release toxins.

- Sit and breathe deeply to eliminate toxins through the lungs. This also helps to calm your nervous system.

- Schedule a massage, reflexology, shiatsu, or other types of bodywork. This helps to increase circulation and aid in the detoxification process.

Detox Alert _____

Fasting should be undertaken by individuals in good health or under the supervision of a medical expert. Pregnant and nursing mothers, individuals who are physically depleted and anorexic, and the elderly should avoid fasting.

- Exercise by walking, yoga, stretching, or any form of gentle movement. Working too hard will only tax your body and work up an appetite.

- Rest as much as possible; by relaxing the body, you can detoxify properly.

- Avoid negative thinking, people, and influences.

- Sit in meditation for 10 minutes every morning and evening.

- Take a walk in the natural beauty of nature.

- Expose your hands and arms to sunlight for 15 to 20 minutes each day.

Humility may not be your strong point, but when your belly has been empty for several days your eyes are opened. Millions of children and adults go to bed hungry each night, the world over. Despite your feelings of emptiness, you know there will always be plenty of food for you to eat, while others are not so lucky. Let this week be a nice time to pause for a moment and reflect on all you have to be grateful for in your life.

Mono-Food Fast

Mono means "one," so only one food should be consumed on fasting days. Although not a total "fast" from solid food, it is less stressful on the body than eating a variety of foods. Your digestive system doesn't have to work as hard to break down one food. It can be a fruit, a vegetable, or a whole grain. Fruits and vegetables should be raw. If you choose to eat a grain during your fast, it can be cooked with plenty of pure water (follow the recipe for brown rice in Chapter 14).

Some schools of thought say the food can be cooked and some say raw only. An alternate version of the Mono-Food Fast is to eat one food, but a different food at each meal: breakfast is apples, lunch is grains, dinner is carrots. This can give you some variety and possibly help you to stay with it a bit longer.

Preparation

If you have a history of eating sweet foods, have the cooked grain or vegetable. Otherwise, a day of fruit can be very healing for the body. Here are three easily digested and nutrient-dense fruits that work well for a Mono-Food Fast:

◆ *Apples:* To keep your blood sugar from spiking, eat only green Granny Smith apples. Have one for each meal or just for breakfast and another fruit for lunch and dinner. You can juice a few as a snack, but dilute by half with distilled water. Apples are a great remedy for constipation due to their high pectin content. One cup of apple juice yields 15 milligrams calcium, 1.5 milligrams iron, 250 milligrams potassium, and 2 milligrams vitamin C.

Pure Insights

There is no other remedial agent or herb in the whole range of known therapeutic agents that can compare with the apple tree and, although it would be difficult to say which of its many virtues is the greatest, we suggest that its abundance of nascent oxygen compound is probably the main reason why it is such a precious food, blood purifier, and unfailing remedy for so many forms of diseases.

—Edward E. Shook, Ph.D., herbologist

◆ *Papaya:* Loaded with enzymes, this tropical fruit helps to reduce inflammation and digestive problems. It can also be used externally for a facial (see Chapter 19). Wash and peel a ripe papaya, then remove the seeds and cut into chunks. Store in the refrigerator in a glass container. Have three small bowls during the day or when hungry. Drink distilled water and peppermint tea in between.

◆ *Grapefruit:* This citrus fruit has become more sweet and seedless over the years. One large grapefruit contains 51 milligrams calcium, 51 milligrams phosphorus, 1.3 milligrams iron, 432 milligrams potassium, 30 International Units (IU) of vitamin A, and 122 milligrams vitamin C. What helps it burn body fat is the white rind on the inside of the skin. This contains bioflavonoids, which help to maintain the small blood capillaries and burn stored fat.

Instructions

Prepare: Days One and Two

Upon rising: The juice of ½ lemon in 8 oz. distilled water. Take a walk, followed by stretching or yoga and deep-breathing exercises.

Breakfast: Bowl of fresh, raw fruit (avoid bananas for their high sugar content).

Lunch: Raw vegetable salad with lemon, garlic, and extra-virgin olive oil dressing.

Dinner: Steamed vegetables with lemon, garlic, and extra-virgin olive oil dressing.

Snack: Between meals have a smoothie made with 8 oz. fresh vegetable juice, 1 TB. flax meal, 1 TB. flaxseed oil, and a green-foods powder (see Chapter 6).

Fast: Days Three and Four

Upon rising: The juice of ½ lemon in 8 oz. distilled water. Take a walk, followed by stretching or yoga and deep-breathing exercises.

Breakfast: 8 oz. fresh fruit juice and/or one Granny Smith apple.

Midmorning: Cup of dandelion tea.

Healthy Tidbits

Fasting is an excellent treatment for autoimmune disease, as it helps to boost the immune system while suppressing overactive immune function.

Lunch: One finely grated medium carrot, sprinkled with fresh lemon juice.

Snack: Cup of herbal tea, such as dandelion, burdock, or nettle.

Dinner: Two boiled red-skinned potatoes. As an option, you can purée the potatoes with the cooking water and eat as a soup.

End Fast: Day Five

Upon rising: The juice of ½ lemon in 8 oz. distilled water.

Breakfast: 1 cup fresh blueberries.

Lunch: Salad of freshly grated cabbage, carrots, and beets tossed with fresh lemon juice.

Snack: 8 oz. fresh vegetable juice.

Dinner: Fresh vegetable salad with lemon, garlic, and extra-virgin olive oil dressing.

Complete: Days Six and Seven

Upon rising: The juice of ½ lemon in 8 oz. distilled water.

Breakfast: ½ cup soft grains, toasted pumpkin seeds, and cooked spinach.

Snack: 8 oz. fresh vegetable juice.

Lunch: Fresh green salad with grilled salmon.

Snack: One raw apple.

Dinner: Miso soup and vegetable brown rice stir-fry.

The Master Cleanse

The Master Cleanse helps to dissolve and eliminate congestion in the form of mucus from your kidneys, digestive system, and liver. Staples of the diet are lemon or lime, rich sources of vitamins and minerals; and pure maple syrup, containing essential nutrients and enough sugar to sustain your energy during the fast. The cayenne pepper is used to break up mucus and provide some warmth to the digestive system.

Lemonade Recipe

Prepare fresh each day. Makes about 8 cups.

8 cups pure water

Juice of 4 fresh lemons or limes

3 TB. pure maple syrup

⅛ tsp. cayenne pepper

Combine ingredients in a large glass jar or pitcher. Drink at room temperature. Drink 6 to 12 cups per day.

Instructions

Prepare: Days One and Two

Upon rising: The juice of ½ lemon in 8 oz. distilled water. Take a walk, followed by stretching or yoga and deep-breathing exercises.

Breakfast: Bowl of fresh, raw fruit or soft nongluten grains.

Lunch: Raw vegetable salad with lemon, garlic, and extra-virgin olive oil dressing.

Dinner: Steamed vegetables with lemon, garlic, and extra-virgin olive oil dressing.

Snack: Between meals have a smoothie made with 8 oz. fresh vegetable juice, 1 TB. flax meal, 1 TB. flaxseed oil, and a green-foods powder (see Chapter 6).

Fast: Days Three and Four

Breakfast: 8 oz. fresh lemonade. Take a walk, followed by stretching or yoga and deep-breathing exercises. Throughout the day drink 6 to 12 glasses of the lemonade.

End Fast: Day Five

Upon rising: 8 oz. fresh lemonade.

Breakfast: One piece of raw organic fruit in season.

Lunch: Salad of freshly grated cabbage, carrots, and beets tossed with fresh lemon juice. This will help your intestines begin moving again.

Snack: 8 oz. fresh lemonade.

Dinner: Fresh vegetable salad or steamed vegetables with lemon, garlic, and extra-virgin olive oil dressing.

Complete: Days Six and Seven

Upon rising: 8 oz. fresh lemonade.

Breakfast: ½ cup soft grains, toasted pumpkin seeds, and cooked spinach.

Snack: 8 oz. fresh vegetable juice.

Lunch: Fresh green salad with grilled salmon.

Snack: One raw apple.

Dinner: Miso soup and vegetable brown rice stir-fry.

Fresh-Juice Fast

Fresh fruit and vegetable juices are excellent choices for those new to the experience of fasting. While water fasting may seem too extreme for your first fast, freshly juiced organic fruits and vegetables can be beneficial and purifying to the body.

In preparation for the fast, for the three days before the fast, begin eating raw fruits and vegetables during the day and eliminate cooked and processed foods. During the fast, drink nothing but distilled water and fresh juices diluted half-and-half with water. All together you will drink 1 cup of diluted fresh vegetable or fruit juice three times a day, as well as herbal tea. In the evening, have some warm soup broth to help warm your body. The whole juice fasting process includes two days to prepare for the fast, one to two days of fasting, and one day to come off the fast.

Detox Alert

Pesticides tend to concentrate in the juice, so juice organic fruits and vegetables only.

Juicing Recipes

There's no need to wonder what combinations of vegetables to use with the following list. Feel free to make up your own juice combinations. To receive the most benefits, drink the juice right after extraction, while still fresh.

- 2 apples, 1 pear, ½ lime

- 2 carrots, handful parsley, handful spinach, 2 stalks celery

- 3 stalks celery, 2 apples, 2-inch piece fresh ginger

- 2 broccoli stalks, fresh rosemary, 2 carrots, ½ lemon

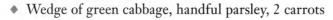

Healthy Tidbits

With all the juicers on the market, buy one with a powerful motor that can juice more than 1 cup at a time. Prices vary, but you can find one for under $100.

- Wedge of green cabbage, handful parsley, 2 carrots

- 3 stalks celery, 2 kale leaves, 1 broccoli stem, 2 carrots

- 1 cup pineapple, 1 apple, ½ lime, 1 slice fresh ginger

You know what you like. Be creative, experiment with combinations, and remember to dilute the juice with distilled water. For superior digestion you will want to "drink your food and chew your liquid," releasing the digestive enzymes in your mouth and giving them plenty of time to do their work.

Instructions

Prepare: Days One and Two

Upon rising: The juice of ½ lemon in 8 oz. distilled water. Take a walk, followed by stretching or yoga and deep-breathing exercises.

Breakfast: Bowl of fresh, raw fruit.

Lunch: Raw vegetable salad with lemon, garlic, and extra-virgin olive oil dressing.

Dinner: Steamed vegetables with lemon, garlic, and extra-virgin olive oil dressing.

Snack: Between meals have a smoothie made with 8 oz. fresh vegetable juice, 1 TB. flax meal, 1 TB. flaxseed oil, and a green-foods powder (see Chapter 6).

Fast: Days Three and Four

Upon rising: The juice of ¹⁄₂ lemon in 8 oz. distilled water. Take a walk, followed by stretching or yoga and deep-breathing exercises.

Breakfast: 8 oz. fresh fruit juice.

Snack: Cup of dandelion tea.

Lunch: 8 oz. fresh vegetable juice.

Snack: Cup of herbal tea, such as dandelion, burdock, or nettle.

Dinner: 8 oz. fresh vegetable juice.

End Fast: Day Five

Upon rising: The juice of ¹⁄₂ lemon in 8 oz. distilled water.

Breakfast: One piece of raw organic fruit.

Lunch: Salad of freshly grated cabbage, carrots, and beets tossed with fresh lemon juice. This will help get your bowels moving again.

Snack: 8 oz. fresh vegetable juice.

Dinner: Fresh vegetable salad with lemon, garlic, and extra-virgin olive oil dressing.

Complete: Day Six and Seven

Upon rising: 8 oz. fresh lemonade.

Breakfast: ¹⁄₂ cup soft grains, toasted pumpkin seeds, and cooked spinach.

Snack: 8 oz. fresh vegetable juice.

Lunch: Fresh green salad with grilled salmon.

Snack: One raw apple.

Dinner: Miso soup and vegetable brown rice stir-fry.

Raw-Food Fast

The Raw-Food Fast consists of eating only raw, uncooked fruits and vegetables for 24 hours or longer. It's a great way to detox your digestive system, and it's perfect for when you cannot juice or fast entirely on liquids. Try doing a day of raw, uncooked foods once a week for better digestive health.

Dressing Ideas

Purchase fruits and vegetables in season and locally grown if possible. You not only support your community farmers, but your body is more in tune with the food in your environment rather than what's been grown 5,000 miles away.

Salads can be creative, satisfying, and delicious. Don't hesitate to experiment and try foods you wouldn't normally eat. Assemble your raw veggies in a bowl, then top with fresh sprouts and one of these delicious dressings.

> **Pure Insights**
>
> If it doesn't have more than 5 ingredients, doesn't take more than 5 minutes to make, and doesn't cost more than $5 for ingredients, I will enjoy it.
>
> —Dr. Doug Graham, chiropractor and raw foods advocate, on the raw-food 5-5-5 rule

Tomato Herb Dressing

2 fresh tomatoes, peeled and quartered

½ garlic clove

½ tsp. each thyme, oregano, rosemary, and basil

Juice of ½ lemon

Purée all ingredients in a blender.

Maple Lemon Dressing

4 TB. flax oil or extra-virgin olive oil

2 TB. fresh lemon juice

½ tsp. maple syrup

2 shakes of *Umeboshi vinegar* (optional)

Mix well and use immediately.

def•i•ni•tion

Umeboshi vinegar is produced from Japanese pickled plums. It has a pink color with a fruity, sour flavor. Technically it is not a vinegar, because it is salty. It works in total harmony with other vinegars and as a salt substitute. It's also very alkalinizing for the blood.

Carrot Ginger Dressing

1 medium carrot

4 TB. flax oil or extra-virgin olive oil

2 green onions, chopped

Juice of ½ lemon

½ tsp. Umeboshi vinegar

1 tsp. ginger juice (grate the ginger and squeeze)

½ cup water

Place ingredients in a blender and purée until smooth. Adjust water for consistency.

≈⌒

Instructions

Prepare: Days One and Two

Upon rising: The juice of ½ lemon in 8 oz. distilled water. Take a walk, followed by stretching or yoga and deep-breathing exercises.

Breakfast: Bowl of fresh, raw fruit.

Lunch: Vegetable salad with lemon, garlic, and extra-virgin olive oil dressing.

Dinner: Steamed vegetables with lemon, garlic, and extra-virgin olive oil dressing.

Snack: Between meals have a smoothie made with 8 oz. fresh vegetable juice, 1 TB. flax meal, 1 TB. flaxseed oil, and a green-foods powder (see Chapter 6).

Fast: Days Three and Four

Upon rising: The juice of ½ lemon in 8 oz. distilled water. Take a walk, followed by stretching or yoga and deep-breathing exercises.

Breakfast: Bowl of fresh, raw fruit.

Snack: Cup of dandelion tea.

Lunch: Raw vegetable salad with choice of dressing.

Snack: Cup of herbal tea, such as dandelion, burdock, or nettle.

Dinner: Raw vegetable salad with your choice of dressing.

Note: Include 8 oz. fresh vegetable juice with meals.

End Fast: Day Five

Upon rising: The juice of ¹/₂ lemon in 8 oz. distilled water.

Breakfast: One piece of raw fruit.

Lunch: Salad of freshly grated cabbage, carrots, and beets tossed with fresh lemon juice.

Snack: 8 oz. fresh vegetable juice.

Dinner: Vegetable salad with lemon, garlic, and extra-virgin olive oil dressing.

Complete: Days Six and Seven

Upon rising: 8 oz. fresh lemonade.

Breakfast: ¹/₂ cup soft grains, toasted pumpkin seeds, and cooked spinach.

Snack: 8 oz. fresh vegetable juice.

Lunch: Fresh green salad with grilled salmon.

Snack: One raw apple.

Dinner: Miso soup and vegetable brown rice stir-fry.

Healthy Tidbits

Your 24-hour fast can begin …

- Upon rising in the morning until following morning.
- From lunch to next day's lunch.
- From dinner to next evening's dinner.

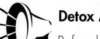

Detox Alert

Before breaking your fast, read Chapter 12 for instructions on how to keep from undoing all your good work.

The Least You Need to Know

◆ Fasting is to intentionally go without food for religious, spiritual, or health reasons.

◆ Although not a total fast from solid food, the Mono-Food Fast can be detoxifying while giving your digestive system a rest.

◆ The Master Cleanse uses fresh lemon or lime juice to dissolve and eliminate congestion from the kidneys, the digestive system, and the liver.

◆ A Fresh-Juice Fast of fruits and vegetables is a good basic fast for individuals fasting for the first time.

◆ A Raw-Food Fast is a great way to detoxify your system when you cannot fast on liquids alone.

12

Week Four: After the Fast

In This Chapter

◆ How to end your fast

◆ Foods to reintroduce

◆ Combining foods for optimal digestion

◆ Your week four shopping checklist

◆ Meals and snacks for week four

How you complete your fast is the most important part of your detox program. You are now lighter and internally cleaner and wondering what you should eat. If you did a short one- to three-day fast, you are probably feeling hungry as well. On longer fasts, after the fourth day, all hunger leaves you and returns when the body needs nutrition in the form of food. For week four you will follow the basic eating plan as outlined in Chapter 10, with a few additions.

In this chapter, you will find instructions for how to break your fast, what foods to reintroduce to your diet, and the benefits of food combining and sea vegetables. Your body is still cleansing and healing, but now on a much deeper level. Let's ease back into eating a wider diet slowly and continue to benefit from your body detoxing.

Breaking the Fast

This is the most important part of your week of fasting. If not done correctly, it can hinder all the good work you have been doing. A sudden return to caffeine, refined sugar, and processed foods would be a terrible shock to your body's systems. Why pour trash down your throat when the house is now clean?

Detox Alert

Take as many days as you fasted to return to a normal diet.

Begin with breakfast on the first day following your fast. Because your stomach has shrunk in size, be careful not to overeat. Have one piece of raw fruit and chew it to liquid.

In between meals have some fresh vegetable juice or lemonade.

For lunch, make a small raw salad of grated carrot, beet, and cabbage tossed with lemon juice. Remember to chew well before swallowing. What a difference this will make for your digestion!

For dinner, lightly steam some vegetables or have another small salad. Dress it with lemon, garlic, and extra-virgin olive oil or another raw-food dressing.

Before bedtime, have a cup of herbal tea and take your probiotics.

Over the next few days, begin to add whole grains, legumes, seeds, animal protein, and nuts. If you add one food at a time you will be able to see if you have a reaction to eating that particular food. This is an important time to listen to your body.

Reintroducing Foods

You may be yearning for a big slice of gooey pizza, but the foods you should re-introduce are much better for you. Another week without flour, sugar, caffeine, and alcohol is your body's idea of a great vacation. You should already have many of the recommended foods in your pantry from before the fast. Stock up on organic fruits and vegetables and follow the menus at the end of this chapter.

Healthy Tidbits

In order to break a habit, an individual must repeat a new habit 500 times before it becomes locked into the psyche. You also have to turn away from the habits you want to break 500 times in order for them to be completely eliminated from your mind and body. In other words, you will need to be patient and persistent to affect the changes you want to see happen.

The foods you will continue to eat represent the superfoods of the earth's bounty. These are nutrient-rich foods that nourish you on a cellular level. They also protect you from developing cancer and disease in general. Detoxing or not, you still want to have these foods as a part of your life-long eating plan.

> **Pure Insights**
>
> Remember, there are no incurable diseases, only people who think they are incurable.
>
> —Dr. John R. Christopher, naturopathic doctor

What You Can Eat

Continue to eat at least five servings of a wide variety of vegetables daily. Have two to three of those servings include kale, collards, spinach, and curly leaf lettuce.

Enjoy modest amounts of the starchy vegetables: winter squash, red-skinned potatoes, corn on the cob, and lima beans.

Continue eating only nonglutinous whole grains: quinoa, millet, brown rice, and amaranth, but include buckwheat.

Have 4 ounces of organic chicken, fish, turkey, or eggs; one or two meals per day.

Use organic beans and legumes as vegetarian protein sources; one or two meals per day.

Eat mildly sweet fruits such as apples, berries, and kiwi; two servings per day.

Drink organic herbal teas: peppermint, spearmint, chamomile, rose hip, licorice root, red clover, dandelion, burdock root, echinacea root, Pau D'arco, nettle, and *kukicha twig*.

Eat soaked or roasted organic seeds in moderation.

> **def•i•ni•tion**
>
> **Kukicha twig** tea is made from roasting the twigs and leaves of the green tea plant. It contains 90 percent less caffeine than regular brewed coffee. Kukicha helps to alkalinize the blood.

Drink lemon, lime, grapefruit, or unsweetened cranberry juice mixed with water.

Use fresh and dried herbs in your cooking. Include raw and cooked garlic with your meals.

Use cold-pressed, organic oils: extra-virgin olive oil, ghee, coconut, and sesame oil for cooking.

Take flaxseed (unheated) and cod liver oil daily.

For sweeteners, use stevia and xylitol.

Drink six to eight glasses of distilled, spring, or filtered water only.

Have freshly made almond milk. Add 1 cup of almonds to a blender with 4 cups of water, 1 teaspoon vanilla extract (optional), and stevia to taste. Purée until well blended (about two to three minutes), strain through cheesecloth, and refrigerate. Lasts four to five days. (Try using other nuts and seeds as well.)

Drink fresh organic vegetable juices daily. Use raw, unfiltered apple cider vinegar as a refreshing health drink. Add 1 teaspoon unrefined apple cider vinegar to 4 ounces of water and sweeten with stevia. Have 30 minutes before a meal to aid digestion and weight loss.

Take the probiotics acidophilus and bifidus morning and night on an empty stomach.

Take one to two digestive enzymes with meals and between meals.

To minimize bowel toxicity and constipation, drink a cup of a light laxative tea before bed at night.

Have a fiber drink in the morning to support healthy bowel function.

Sea Vegetables

Sea vegetables are commonly and incorrectly referred to as seaweed. These super-foods are often overlooked in Western diets but are a diet staple in Asian countries. In *Healing with Whole Foods* (see Appendix D), researcher Paul Pitchford lists the general properties of sea vegetables:

- Soften hardened areas and masses in the body
- Help to detoxify
- Moisten dryness
- Act as a diuretic
- Remove residues of radiation from the body
- Improve water metabolism
- Act as lymphatic cleansers
- Alkalize the blood
- Activate liver energy
- Are beneficial to the thyroid
- Help lower cholesterol

Compared to milk, sea vegetables have up to 10 times more calcium and up to eight times more iron than beef. They supply iodine, fluorine, and B vitamins in an absorbable form. The sea vegetables dulse, nori, arame, kombu, wakame, and hijiki

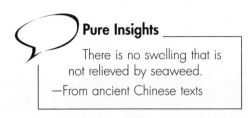

Pure Insights

There is no swelling that is not relieved by seaweed.
—From ancient Chinese texts

are sold in the local health food store or oriental market. They require presoaking and cooking, but are delicious served in soups, salads, or as a side dish.

If you have eaten in a Japanese restaurant, you will have tasted sea vegetables. Nori would have been used to wrap sushi; wakame flavors the miso soup; and the seaweed salad is an assortment of sea vegetables tossed with a sesame-flavored dressing. I suggest you check online to explore the numerous recipes and books for preparing these nutritious foods.

Food Combining

Combining your foods for optimal digestion has a long and controversial history, which continues to this day. It is a simple and easy premise that is best experienced to understand how it works. Basically, foods are separated into groups that require a particular enzyme for digestive purposes. These can be an acidic gastric juice or alkaline pancreatic enzymes. When several types of food are eaten together, the necessary gastric juices and enzymes compete with one another, which compromises digestion in the stomach.

Protein foods depend on gastric acid, which consists of hydrochloric acid and an acidic enzyme called pepsin.

Fats are emulsified by bile, and carbohydrates require pancreatic enzymes and are mostly broken down in the small intestine.

Because enzymes decline as we age, heartburn and indigestion become more prevalent. We can help to alleviate these symptoms by eating more raw foods high in natural enzymes, following food combining guidelines, and/or taking digestive enzyme supplements with meals.

Food-combining guidelines take some getting used to, but are easy to remember. Don't worry if you cannot always follow them exactly. If you manage the majority of the time, you will notice a positive difference in your digestion and in your ability to lose unwanted weight.

♦ Fruits digest in 45 minutes, so eat them alone and on an empty stomach. If eaten with protein or grains they can ferment, slow down digestion, and cause intestinal gas.

♦ Animal protein digests in six to eight hours. Combine with easily digested non-starchy vegetables and sea vegetables.

♦ Grains and starchy vegetables digest in four to six hours. These include all whole grains, dry cereals, and flour products plus winter squash, potatoes, peas, corn, lima beans, water chestnuts, artichokes, and Jerusalem artichokes. Eat them with nonstarchy vegetables and sea vegetables.

♦ Large amounts of fat and fried foods delay the secretion of hydrochloric acid needed to digest protein. Avoid combining a large amount of fat with a protein food. Burping is your signal that oil and protein don't mix.

To sum it up, avoid eating protein (steak) and starch (potato) together, or chicken and rice. Eat them separately and with lots of raw and cooked vegetables. Make 80 percent of the food on your plate cooked and raw vegetables. The remaining 20 percent can be protein or grains and starchy vegetables.

Week Four Shopping Checklist

FRUITS:

❑ Lemons

❑ Limes

❑ Peaches

❑ Granny Smith apples

❑ Strawberries

❑ Pineapple

❑ Blueberries

❑ Pears

❑ Raisins

VEGETABLES:

❑ Spinach (fresh or frozen)

❑ Baby spinach

❑ Arugula

❑ Watercress

❑ Mesclun salad greens

❑ Red leaf lettuce

❑ Kale

❑ Escarole

❑ Asparagus

❑ Broccoli rabe

❑ Broccoli

❏ Carrots

❏ Celery

❏ Beets

❏ Fennel bulbs

❏ Onions

❏ Red onions

❏ Green onions

❏ Garlic

❏ Green beans

❏ Spaghetti squash

❏ Snow peas

❏ Cabbage

❏ Cucumber

❏ Wild mushrooms

❏ Tomatoes

❏ Zucchini

❏ Red peppers

LIQUIDS AND BEVERAGES:

❏ Dandelion tea

❏ Chamomile tea

❏ Rice milk

❏ Distilled or filtered water

❏ Tomato juice

❏ Coconut milk

❏ Cranberry juice (unsweetened)

❏ Vegetable stock

SWEETENERS:

❏ Stevia

❏ Xylitol

OILS AND CONDIMENTS:

❏ Apple cider vinegar

❏ Extra-virgin olive oil

❏ White miso

❏ Fiber powder

❏ Flax meal

❏ Flaxseed oil

❏ Sesame oil

❏ Rice vinegar

❏ Butter

❏ Sea salt

SEEDS:

❏ Sunflower

❏ Pumpkin

❏ Pine nuts

❏ Tahini (sesame butter)

HERBS AND SPICES:

❏ Ginger

❏ Parsley

❏ Cayenne pepper

❏ Dill

❏ Basil

❏ Cinnamon

❏ Curry

❏ Cumin

❏ Turmeric

PROTEIN:

❑ Wild salmon

❑ Tilapia

❑ Halibut

❑ Chicken

❑ Lamb

❑ Extra-firm tofu

❑ Eggs

❑ Edamame (frozen soy beans)

GRAINS:

❑ Cream of rice cereal

❑ Quinoa

❑ Short-grain brown rice

❑ Mochi (plain and cinnamon raisin)

BEANS:

❑ Cannellini

❑ Chickpeas

❑ Black beans

❑ Lentils

SEA VEGETABLES:

❑ Arame

PREPARED FOOD:

❑ Vegetarian chili

❑ Dolmades (stuffed grape leaves)

❑ Hummus

❑ Marinara sauce

Week Four Meals and Snacks

Menus for week four are repeated from week two with a few new additions. This gives you the opportunity to use up the foods you bought in week two. Have stevia and xylitol for your sweeteners. Continue to avoid flour, sugar, caffeine, alcohol, and pasteurized fruit juice for one more week.

Day One

Upon rising: The juice of ½ lemon in 8 oz. water, sweetened with stevia; fiber powder or 1 TB. flax meal in water (can also be added to a fruit smoothie).

Breakfast: Cream of rice cereal; fresh strawberries; 1 TB. sunflower seeds.

Snack: One Granny Smith apple.

Lunch: Grilled lamb; asparagus; garlic-sautéed broccoli rabe; salad greens, grated carrots and beets with Tahini Lemon Dressing (see recipe in Appendix B).

Snack: Toasted pumpkin seeds and raisins.

Dinner: Miso soup with sliced carrots, green onions, and white miso; Arame and Brown Rice (see recipe in Appendix B); cooked greens and black beans; fresh green salad with apple cider vinegar, garlic, and olive oil.

Before bedtime: The juice of ½ lemon in 8 oz. water, sweetened with stevia. Take your probiotics.

Day Two

Upon rising: The juice of ½ lemon in 8 oz. water, sweetened with stevia; fiber powder or 1 TB. flax meal in water.

Breakfast: Organic eggs; cooked spinach; plain mochi.

Snack: Fresh vegetable juice: in a juice extractor, process until smooth 2 carrots, 3-inch piece ginger, and 1 apple.

Lunch: Arugula, mesclun, and watercress salad with wild salmon.

Snack: Pineapple Coconut Smoothie: purée in a blender 1 cup fresh pineapple, ¼ cup unsweetened coconut milk, and 1 cup rice milk. Sweeten with stevia to taste.

Dinner: Steamed spaghetti squash with marinara sauce and cannellini beans; fresh green salad with fennel, red onion, and garlic lemon dressing.

Before bedtime: Cup of dandelion tea. Take your probiotics.

Day Three

Upon rising: The juice of ½ lemon in 8 oz. water, sweetened with stevia; fiber powder or 1 TB. flax meal in water.

Breakfast: Apple Strawberry Smoothie: purée in a blender ½ green apple, 8 strawberries, and a scoop of fiber powder. Sweeten with stevia to taste.

Snack: 1 hard-boiled egg; tomato juice.

Lunch: Baked tilapia; green beans; quinoa tossed with sautéed garlic; fresh mesclun salad.

Dinner: Vegetarian chili over brown rice; fresh spinach salad.

Before bedtime: The juice of ½ lemon in 8 oz. water, sweetened with stevia. Take your probiotics.

Day Four

Upon rising: The juice of ½ lemon in 8 oz. water, sweetened with stevia; fiber powder or 1 TB. flax meal in water.

Breakfast: Soft Brown Rice and Quinoa (see recipe in Appendix B).

Snack: One ripe peach.

Lunch: Spinach and salmon salad (toss together green onions, baby spinach, cooked snow peas, sesame oil, rice vinegar, Umeboshi vinegar, and lime juice; top with grilled salmon).

Snack: Fresh vegetable juice: in a juice extractor, process until smooth 2 carrots, ¼ beet, 2 stalks of celery, and a handful of parsley.

Dinner: Hummus platter with grilled vegetables; dolmades (stuffed grape leaves); green salad.

Before bed: Cup of chamomile tea. Take your probiotics.

Day Five

Upon rising: The juice of ½ lemon in 8 oz. water, sweetened with stevia; fiber powder or 1 TB. flax meal in water.

Breakfast: Eggs Florentine (see recipe in Appendix B).

Snack: Two kiwis.

Lunch: Edamame, red onion, grated carrots, and cooked broccoli tossed with olive oil and apple cider vinegar, topped with toasted pine nuts, on mesclun greens.

Snack: Fresh vegetable juice: in a juice extractor, process until smooth 2 carrots, 3 celery stalks, small wedge of cabbage, and ½ cucumber.

Dinner: Risotto with Wild Mushrooms (see recipe in Appendix B).

Before bedtime: The juice of ½ lemon in 8 oz. water, sweetened with stevia. Take your probiotics.

Day Six

Upon rising: The juice of ½ lemon in 8 oz. water, sweetened with stevia; fiber powder or 1 TB. flax meal in water.

Breakfast: Vegetable omelet; cinnamon raisin mochi.

Snack: One apple.

Lunch: Roasted Salmon with Lemon Garlic Sauce (see recipes in Appendix B).

Snack: Fresh vegetable juice: in a juice extractor, process until smooth 2 carrots, 3 stalks celery, 2 tomatoes, 4 spinach leaves, and 4 kale leaves. Pour juice into a blender and add 3 sprigs dill, juice of 1 lemon, 1 clove garlic, ½ tsp. cayenne pepper, and 1 tsp. Umeboshi vinegar. Purée until smooth.

Dinner: Quinoa Lettuce Wraps (see recipe in Appendix B); lentil vegetable soup.

Before bedtime: Cup of dandelion tea. Take your probiotics.

Day Seven

Upon rising: The juice of ½ lemon in 8 oz. water, sweetened with stevia; fiber powder or 1 TB. flax meal in water.

Breakfast: Mochi waffles with cinnamon/stevia sprinkle (in a shaker container combine 4 parts cinnamon to 1 part stevia powder and mix well); butter; fresh blueberries.

Snack: One pear.

Lunch: Vegetable Shish Kabobs (see recipe in Appendix B); fresh vegetable salad.

Snack: Fresh vegetable juice: in a juice extractor, process until smooth ½ cucumber, 2 carrots, 1 apple, and the juice of ½ lemon.

Dinner: Stir-fried vegetables with chicken; cooked quinoa; fresh green salad.

Before bedtime: The juice of ½ lemon in 8 oz. water, sweetened with stevia. Take your probiotics.

The Least You Need to Know

◆ It's important to return to eating whole foods gradually so that your digestive system can adapt to the change.

◆ In week four, continue to eliminate flour, sugar, caffeine, and alcohol while your body continues to detoxify following the fast.

◆ The nutrient-rich foods you are eating will nourish you on a cellular level, protect you from disease, and should be a part of your life-long eating plan.

◆ Sea vegetables have up to 10 times more calcium and up to 8 times more iron than beef and supply iodine, fluorine, and B vitamins in an absorbable form.

◆ Food combining separates food into groups that require either an acidic gastric juice or an alkaline pancreatic enzyme for digestive purposes.

13

Week Five: A New Lifestyle

In This Chapter

- ◆ Your lifetime eating plan
- ◆ Keeping a balanced blood pH
- ◆ The satisfying five flavors: sweet, sour, bitter, pungent, and salty
- ◆ Take time to occasionally trash and cleanse
- ◆ Your week five shopping checklist
- ◆ Meals and snacks for week five

It's time to go back to the questionnaire in Chapter 1 and reanswer the questions based on how you are feeling now. Add up the numbers and compare them to the numbers from four weeks ago. Have they changed at all? Have any of your symptoms eased up or disappeared completely?

Changing how and what you eat can be a difficult undertaking. Actually, change of any kind is not easy. There is comfort in holding on to what we know, even if it is harmful to us. The unknown is daunting, and uncharted territory. Your mind will produce a million excuses why you should not change what you eat. Listen to the excuses, write them down, and realize they are only excuses. Then write a list of the benefits you have gotten from doing the detox program. It will speak for itself.

In this chapter, you will find your lifetime eating plan. You'll learn about balancing an acid/alkaline blood pH and how to satisfy your body with the five flavors. You are ready to take on a dietary lifestyle designed to keep you active and healthy. You experienced the lifetime eating plan in week one of your detox (see Chapter 9). You've already prepared and tasted the foods, and some of them are in your pantry and freezer. You've come full circle and now find yourself at the perfect place to live.

Where to Go From Here

You won't have to change much now that you know how good you feel eating a whole-foods diet. I suggest you stay where you are and add back a few foods I list later in the chapter. Because of the difficulty in digesting dairy, refined sugar, and wheat products, keep them out of your diet or have them on rare occasions. You now know you can live just fine without them.

When you do eat dairy products, have small amounts made from goat or sheep's milk. Goat's milk has less fat and milk sugar than cow's milk, but is higher in fatty acids. This makes it easier for you to digest. Feta, chevre, and Romano cheeses can be found in your grocery store made from goat or sheep's milk.

Wheat can now be found in all processed-food products, which is encouragement enough to prepare your own meals. When you eat out, avoid having bread with meals. Keep only wheat-free whole-grain breads and pastas at home, and you won't feel deprived.

Sugar is the leading cause of health problems in the world. It is addictive and deadly for all your body's systems. There was a time when sugar was only eaten at special occasions like weddings and holidays. Today it is a major component of America's diet, and we can see the results in the high levels of obesity, diabetes, heart, and auto-immune disease.

When you read labels, look for the names that mean sugar:

- Corn syrup
- Maltose
- Dextrose
- Glucose
- Cane sugar or crystals
- Fructose
- Barley malt
- Rice syrup
- Fruit juice concentrate
- Brown sugar

Continue to use the herbal sweeteners stevia and xylitol, and enjoy natural sweeteners—honey, maple, rice, and agave syrups—on occasion.

To maintain adequate dietary fiber, take 2 to 3 tablespoons of ground flax meal daily. This also provides valuable omega-3 fatty acids and aids in weight loss.

Complete your last meal no later than 7:30 P.M., leaving time for digestion.

Maintain a daily exercise program that fits your lifestyle.

Periodically have a relaxing massage, and continue to include sauna and/or steam baths in your health regimen.

Most important is to plan and prepare foods ahead of time. You can wash and dry two to three days' worth of salad greens and store them in the refrigerator. Also, make and freeze several sauces ahead of time. You can use them when you need a quick topping for grains or vegetables.

I suggest you purchase a good slow cooker and use it regularly. It allows for minimum cooking effort with maximum results. All you have to do is assemble the recipe and turn the slow cooker on—basic and simple. Make a big pot of soup and freeze part of it for those times you don't want to cook. Add a salad and whole-grain bread for a nutritious meal.

Keep on hand half a dozen hard-boiled eggs to use in salads, soups, or for snacks.

Toast or soak a variety of nuts and seeds to have on hand.

Hopefully, these last four weeks have given you some insight into changing your diet and health for the better. If you continue to eat a whole-foods diet as outlined in these chapters, your health will continue to improve as your immune system strengthens.

> **Healthy Tidbits**
>
> Now that you have your juicer up and running, make it part of your routine to drink a glass of fresh organic vegetable juice every day. Use it as a savory afternoon smoothie or quick meal replacement. It is delicious and loaded with easily absorbed nutrients.

> **Pure Insights**
>
> Men should eat more oatmeal. It contains the complex carbohydrates needed to sustain energy and the soluble fiber to lower cholesterol, which clogs blood vessels and contributes to heart disease and erectile dysfunction (impotence).
>
> —James J. Kenney, Ph.D., R.D., nutrition research specialist at Pritikin Longevity Center

Acid/Alkaline Balance

In nature there exist acid foods with an acid pH and alkaline foods with an alkaline pH. There are also foods that change and become acid or alkaline when digested. The ideal blood pH of 7.4 is alkaline. Acid is distinguished by a sour taste and the ability to dissolve metal and neutralize alkaline substances. Research has shown that disease thrives in an acidic environment. Eating a diet high in alkaline-forming foods, particularly fruits and vegetables, helps create the ideal blood pH.

> **Pure Insights** _____
>
> Hydrochloric (HCL) acid is the only acid the body produces. All other acids are by-products of metabolism and are eliminated as soon as possible. HCL keeps us alive by maintaining proper alkaline/acid balance. It then becomes alkaline after its vital job in the digestive process is over.
>
> —Dr. Theodore A. Baroody, *Alkalize or Die*

Animal products, beans, and rice are acid-forming foods, while fruit and most vegetables are alkaline-forming foods. Although lemons, limes, and apple cider vinegar taste acidic, they create an alkaline condition in the body and help reduce body acids. Eighty percent of your meal should consist of alkaline-forming foods, while 20 percent will consist of acid-forming foods. When you look at your plate, the majority of the foods should be cooked and raw vegetables, with the remaining foods grains and/ or animal protein. Continue to take a digestive enzyme with meals and snacks.

Getting the Five Flavors

How many times have you completed a big meal and felt that something was missing? A food, a taste, something your taste buds did not get? Satisfying your taste buds is a very important aspect of preparing a meal. If that one flavor is missing, you will go looking for it in a dessert, coffee, or a late-night snack. The five flavors you want to have in a meal are sweet, sour, bitter, pungent, and salty:

◆ *Sweet* flavor both energizes and relaxes the body. It comes from sweet vegetables such as carrots, onions, cabbage, winter squash, sweet potatoes, fennel, and beets.

◆ *Sour* flavor causes contraction in tissues and has an astringent effect. It can be found in citrus juice, vinegars, cranberries, sauerkraut, and pickles.

- *Bitter* flavor helps with constipation and has a purgative effect. It is found in the green leafy vegetables like kale, arugula, collards, spinach, chicory, and lettuce. Seeking a bitter taste, people often turn to coffee and chocolate. Eat more greens instead.

- *Pungent* flavor stimulates circulation of energy and blood. It comes from garlic, ginger, horseradish, mint, hot chiles, green onions, basil, mustard, and white and black pepper.

> **Pure Insights**
>
> Each day the sweet flavor—the primary flavor of most carbohydrates such as grains, vegetables, legumes, nuts, seeds, and fruit—should be accompanied by small amounts of bitter, salty, pungent, and sour foods.
> —Paul Pitchford, *Healing with Whole Foods*

- *Salty* flavor is used for pain, abdominal swelling, improving digestion, and detoxifying the bowels. Find it in sea salt, sea vegetables, tamari soy sauce, miso, pickles, and umeboshi plum.

Having all five flavors in a meal creates balance and a sense of satisfaction. According to Chinese physiology, the dominant flavor is sweet. Your body is nourished by the sweet flavor, but for balance your meal must include the four other flavors as well.

Staying on Track

You should be feeling pretty good after your detox. You're probably being careful not to eat any foods from the avoid list, hoping to hold on to this good feeling. That is, until you have to attend a wedding, a family holiday, or go on vacation. Naturally you end up having some dessert, alcohol, and bread, and before long, these foods are back in your daily diet. If you can catch it early enough, a brief trashing won't set you back. You can easily move from trashing to cleansing by turning to this chapter and getting back on your lifetime program. Really, it's that simple. The all-American way is to trash and put on weight and then detox by going on a two-week diet. We've been doing this for decades. Weight-loss diets are really our attempt to detoxify the liver and intestines.

> **Detox Alert**
>
> Be careful when adding back sugar, wheat, dairy, or alcohol to your diet. You could have an adverse reaction if you suddenly return to eating them in excess.

According to the Organic Consumers Association, by choosing to eat fruit, beans, vegetables, and whole grains each day over having a small serving of beef, one egg, and a 1-ounce serving of cheese, you would …

- ◆ Increase your daily consumption of dietary fiber by 16 grams. This is more than half the recommended intake.

- ◆ Reduce your intake of fat by 22 grams. This is one third of the recommended daily limit.

- ◆ Reduce your saturated fat by 12 grams. This is more than half the recommended limit.

- ◆ Spare the need for 1.8 acres of cropland, 40 pounds of fertilizer, and 3 ounces of pesticides each year.

- ◆ Dump 11,400 fewer pounds of animal manure into the environment each year.

It is the small changes we make that have a huge impact on our health and our environment. With each day you spend eating nutrient-rich foods, your health will improve, your skin will glow, your eyes will shine, and you will look younger and have more energy than you ever thought possible. Detoxing your body is just the beginning of a whole new life.

Week Five Shopping Checklist

FRUITS:

❑ Lemons

❑ Blueberries (both fresh and frozen)

❑ Apples

❑ Bananas

❑ Red grapes

❑ Strawberries

❑ Pears

❑ Kiwis

❑ Pomegranates

❑ Peaches (frozen)

❑ Raisins

❑ Dried cranberries (sweetened with fruit juice)

VEGETABLES:

❑ Spinach

❑ Arugula

❑ Watercress

❑ Mesclun salad mix

❑ Lettuce

❑ Bok choy

❑ Carrots

❑ Celery

❑ Red onions

❑ Green onions

❑ Sweet onions

❑ Garlic

❑ Kale

❑ Fennel bulbs

❑ Broccoli

❑ Broccoli rabe

❑ Green beans

❑ Asparagus

❑ Tomatoes

❑ Zucchini

❑ Baby bella mushrooms

❑ Red peppers

❑ Jalapeño peppers

❑ Avocadoes

BEVERAGES:

❑ Soy/rice milk

❑ Cranberry juice (unsweetened)

❑ Apple juice

❑ Tomato juice

❑ Distilled or filtered water

❑ Sleepytime tea (a type of tea made by Celestial Seasonings)

❑ Dandelion tea

❑ Camomile tea

❑ Rooibos tea

❑ Coconut milk

SWEETENERS:

❑ Raw honey

❑ Stevia

❑ Maple syrup

OILS AND CONDIMENTS:

❑ Extra-virgin olive oil

❑ Coconut oil

❑ Balsamic vinegar

❑ Vegenaise

❑ Apple cider vinegar

❑ White miso

❑ Sea salt

❑ Salsa

NUTS AND SEEDS:

❑ Almonds

❑ Walnuts

❑ Pumpkin seeds

❑ Pecans

❑ Almond butter

❑ Flax meal

❑ Fiber powder

HERBS AND SPICES:

❑ Fresh basil

❑ Fresh parsley

❑ Ginger root

❑ Cayenne pepper

❑ Cinnamon

PROTEIN:

❑ Wild salmon

❑ Sea scallops

❑ Shrimp

❑ Turkey burgers

❑ Turkey sausage

❑ Chicken breasts

❑ Steak

❑ Lamb chops

❑ Hemp protein powder

❑ Firm tofu

❑ Eggs

GRAINS:

❑ Cream of rice cereal

❑ Buckwheat pancake mix

❑ Steel-cut oatmeal

❑ Wheat-free waffles

❑ Wheat-free hamburger buns

❑ Spelt crackers

❑ Spelt tortillas

❑ Spelt bread

❑ Wild rice

❑ Short-grain brown rice

❑ Spelt angel hair pasta

❑ Brown rice pasta

EXTRAS:

❑ Soy yogurt

❑ Butter

❑ Probiotics

❑ Wooden shish kabob skewers

Week Five Meals and Snacks

In week five you settle into the lifetime eating plan as explained in week one (see Chapter 9). Lemon water continues to be a great beginning for your day, sweetened with xylitol or stevia. Enjoy the adventure of exploring new tastes, new foods, and the physical feelings of well-being that they bring to your body.

Day One

Upon rising: The juice of ½ lemon in 8 oz. water, sweetened with stevia; fiber powder or 1 TB. flax meal in water.

Breakfast: Buckwheat pancakes with organic blueberries and maple syrup; tea or decaffeinated coffee with nondairy milk.

Snack: Spelt crackers or an apple with almond butter.

Lunch: Turkey burger on wheat-free bun with lettuce, tomato, onion, 1 tsp. Vegenaise mixed with 2 tsp. salsa; arugula mesclun salad with balsamic vinegar and olive oil dressing.

Snack: Fresh blueberries or handful of toasted almonds.

Dinner: Broiled or grilled salmon; spelt angel-hair pasta tossed with garlic sautéed in olive oil; steamed broccoli topped with toasted walnuts.

Before bedtime: The juice of ½ lemon in 8 oz. water, sweetened with stevia. Take your probiotics.

Day Two

Upon rising: The juice of ½ lemon in 8 oz. water, sweetened with stevia; fiber powder or 1 TB. flax meal in water.

Breakfast: Veggie omelet with spelt toast and butter; rooibos tea with rice milk and honey.

Snack: Toasted pumpkin seeds with raisins.

Lunch: Mixed-green salad with baked tofu or grilled chicken; vegetable soup; spelt bread with almond butter.

Snack: Banana Apple Smoothie: purée in blender 1 frozen banana; half an organic apple, chopped; 1 cup apple juice or water; ½ tsp. cinnamon; and 1 TB. hemp protein powder. Sweeten to taste.

Dinner: Broccoli rabe and turkey sausage; wild rice topped with toasted almonds; fresh green salad.

Before bedtime: The juice of ½ lemon in 8 oz. water, sweetened with stevia. Take your probiotics.

Day Three

Upon rising: The juice of ½ lemon in 8 oz. water, sweetened with stevia; fiber powder or 1 TB. flax meal in water.

Breakfast: Blueberry Fruit Smoothie: purée in a blender 8 oz. water, 1 TB. hemp protein powder, 1 TB. flax meal, 1 tsp. fiber powder, and ½ cup frozen blueberries; sweeten to taste.

Snack: Tofu Nut Butter (see recipe in Appendix B) on spelt crackers.

Lunch: Roasted vegetables and sliced, grilled chicken rolled-up in a spelt tortilla with Vegenaise; fresh green salad.

Snack: Coconut Ginger Smoothie: purée in blender ¼ cup apple juice; ¼ cup unsweetened coconut milk; ½ banana; ¼ tsp. fresh ginger root, peeled; and ½ cup crushed ice or 2 small ice cubes. Sweeten to taste.

Dinner: Grilled Chicken with Pesto (see recipe in Appendix B); pan-grilled asparagus; water-cooked kale; green salad with lemon–olive oil vinaigrette.

Before bedtime: Unsweetened cranberry juice and water, sweetened with stevia. Take your probiotics.

Day Four

Upon rising: The juice of ½ lemon in 8 oz. water, sweetened with stevia; fiber powder or 1 TB. flax meal in water.

Breakfast: Bowl of steel-cut oatmeal topped with fresh blueberries.

Snack: Sliced kiwis.

Lunch: Watercress Mesclun Salad (see recipe in Appendix B).

Snack: Spicy Vegetable Smoothie: purée in blender 1 cup organic tomato juice; ¼ avocado; ½ tsp. jalapeño pepper, chopped; ¼ tsp. dried cayenne pepper; ¼ cup chopped onion; ½ cup chopped parsley; and 2 cloves garlic, peeled.

Dinner: Grilled salmon, green beans sautéed with onions and garlic; fresh spinach salad.

Before bedtime: Unsweetened cranberry juice and water, sweetened with stevia. Take your probiotics.

Day Five

Upon rising: The juice of ½ lemon in 8 oz. water, sweetened with stevia; fiber powder or 1 TB. flax meal in water.

Breakfast: Wheat-free waffles with fresh blueberries and maple syrup.

Snack: Fresh pear with unsweetened soy yogurt, topped with cinnamon and drizzled with maple syrup.

Lunch: Grilled chicken on spelt bread, with lettuce, tomato, and Vegenaise; fresh spinach salad.

Snack: Raisins; fruit juice–sweetened cranberries; walnuts.

Dinner: Garlic sautéed shrimp; wheat-free rice pasta and fresh tomato sauce; steamed vegetable medley; mesclun salad with lemon-garlic dressing.

Before bedtime: Cup of dandelion tea. Take your probiotics.

Day Six

Upon rising: The juice of ½ lemon in 8 oz. water, sweetened with stevia; fiber powder or 1 TB. flax meal in water.

Breakfast: Poached eggs with cooked spinach; wheat-free toast and butter.

Snack: Sliced strawberries with unsweetened soy yogurt, drizzled with maple syrup.

Lunch: Sliced steak or chicken with avocado; arugula; watercress salad and lemon–olive oil dressing.

Snack: Cooked brown rice mixed with diced carrot, celery, and red onion; tossed with olive oil and lemon juice or apple cider vinegar.

Dinner: Rosemary Balsamic Chicken Kabobs; Watercress Pomegranate Salad (see recipes in Appendix B).

Before bedtime: Cup of chamomile tea. Take your probiotics.

Day Seven

Upon rising: The juice of ½ lemon in 8 oz. water, sweetened with stevia; fiber powder or 1 TB. flax meal in water.

Breakfast: Cream of rice cereal with maple syrup and fresh blueberries.

Snack: Handful of grapes.

Lunch: Grilled lamb chops; Kale Walnut Salad (see recipe in Appendix B).

Snack: Peachy Smoothie: purée in blender 1 cup frozen peach slices; ½ banana, sliced; 3 TB. unsweetened soy yogurt; ¼ cup apple juice; and ½ cup rice milk. Sweeten to taste.

Dinner: Grilled scallops; cooked brown rice tossed with sautéed garlic; grilled asparagus; fresh green salad.

Before bedtime: The juice of ½ lemon in 8 oz. water, sweetened with stevia. Take your probiotics.

The Least You Need to Know

♦ Maintain your healthy diet by staying dairy-, wheat-, and sugar-free.

♦ Save time and effort by planning your meals ahead of time.

♦ Eating a diet high in alkaline-forming foods helps to create the ideal blood pH.

♦ Satisfy your taste buds by featuring the five flavors—sweet, sour, bitter, pungent, and salty—in your diet.

♦ If you get off track on occasion, just return to your lifetime-eating plan to cleanse your system and restore balance.

Part **4**

Alternative Detox Choices

Upon completing the five-week detox program, you can now see how necessary it is to include periodic detoxification as part of a healthy lifestyle. Once you have been eating a whole-foods diet on a regular basis, you can try shorter detox programs. These can be very effective for targeting particular organs and/or health concerns you may be having.

In the next five chapters, you will learn how to detoxify according to the change of seasons, how a weekend fast can feel rejuvenating, and how you can target specific body systems to help you achieve and maintain optimal health.

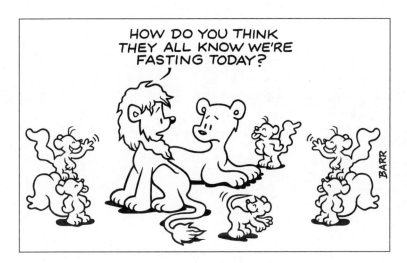

14

Detox for Every Season

In This Chapter

- ◆ Detoxing with the seasons
- ◆ The five elements of nature
- ◆ Planning a spring detox
- ◆ Summertime detox is hot!
- ◆ Purify the system with an autumn detox
- ◆ Whole-grain winter detox

Detoxing with the change of seasons brings one phase of life to an end and prepares you for another. According to Chinese physiology, seasonal changes can affect your health and well-being in profound ways. In ancient China, the change of climate corresponded to the five elements: Fire, Earth, Metal, Water, and Wood. All of life is influenced by these five natural phenomena, including our emotions, body parts, internal organs, and environment. It is knowing how to work within the cycles of nature that can keep you healthy and, ultimately, happy.

In this chapter, you will find the appropriate detox program for each season of the year. You will learn what foods to use and how each season affects you according to the five elements of nature.

Four Times a Year

Early medical doctors saw the "whole" person as an interconnected flow of energy between organs, tissues, and functioning systems in the body. This included the mental and emotional aspects of the individual as well. When one organ is stagnant, it affects another organ, which in turn affects something else, resulting in physical imbalance. Returning harmony to the body requires a balance of nutrients and energy feeding all the systems.

> **Pure Insights** _____
>
> Just as the life of the individual is composed of seasons, the spring of new ideas, the summer of work, the autumn of completion, and the winter of rest and contemplation, so too worldly events have their seasons. When attempting to determine the tendency of a situation, approach it with the predictable plan of the seasons in mind. By contemplating the present situation and taking note of what immediately preceded it, you should be able to determine what will follow.
>
> —R. L. Wing, *I Ching, Book of Changes* (the Chinese book of divination)

As you move from one season to another, take note of what preceded it to know what will follow. The predictable movement of spring into summer; summer into fall; fall into winter; and winter into spring brings a change not only with the weather, but with the food and exercise your body will need. When you observe these natural transitions with an awareness of your body, you will know how to keep yourself healthy.

When shopping for the most appropriate foods for your detox, buy locally grown organic produce in season whenever possible. These foods represent the energetics of a particular season and its climate. Eating tropical bananas in January in New Jersey makes no sense to your body. Tropical foods serve a purpose in the heat and humidity of the tropics. They work at cross purposes to your body in the freezing winter temperatures.

The Five Element Theory

Through observation and study, the ancient Chinese created the Five Element theory, to interpret the relationship between the human body and the natural environment. These five elements—Fire, Earth, Metal, Water, and Wood—represent all aspects of the material world. They connect the complex movement and flow between our physical, emotional, and mental selves with the world around us. By comparing that which was similar to specific reactions and events, these ancient medical practitioners were able to attribute specific phenomenon to each of the elements.

The ancient Chinese then created categories for each element to correspond with these phenomenon. For example, the Wood element represents the liver-gallbladder, with the following qualities:

- Color: green
- Taste: sour
- Sense: sight
- Emotion: anger

- Season: spring
- Direction: east
- Sense organ: eyes

I have listed seven, but the category list is extensive and all-inclusive of these material phenomenon.

According to the Five Element theory, your organs function within the biorhythm cycle of the body and have a peak time during each day when they are the most active. If you tend to consistently awaken each night at 2 A.M., it can signal that your liver may need the support of certain nutrients. It can also do with a good detoxing. It's better to treat an organ during the corresponding season and/or its particular time of day, listed here for each organ based on traditional Chinese medical practices:

> **Healthy Tidbits**
>
> The Five Element theory includes two cycles of balance. One generates and supports (harmonious health): Wood feeds Fire; Fire creates Earth; Earth bears Metal; Metal collects Water; Water nourishes Wood. One overcomes and destroys (disease and illness): Wood parts Earth; Earth absorbs Water; Water quenches Fire; Fire melts Metal; Metal chops Wood.

1–3 A.M.: Liver

3–5 A.M.: Lungs

5–7 A.M.: Colon

7–9 A.M.: Stomach

9–11 A.M.: Spleen/Pancreas

11 A.M.–1 P.M.: Heart

1–3 P.M.: Small Intestines

3–5 P.M.: Bladder

5–7 P.M.: Kidney/Adrenal

7–9 P.M.: Reproductive

9–11 P.M.: Endocrine

11 P.M.–1 A.M.: Gallbladder

With this information, you can plan your detox to correspond with a particular season of the year to better support a specific organ. Coupled with the highest-quality foods, herbs, and supplements, you can use the five elements to heal and rebalance your internal systems. As always, before beginning a detoxification program, consult your medical doctor and continue to have any medications monitored.

Spring Liver Detox

Spring brings us out of the heaviness of winter into longer days, new growth, and endless possibility. The Wood element represents spring. The primary organ influenced is the liver; the secondary organ, the gallbladder. Known as the "General" in Chinese medicine, your liver regulates the movement of vital energy and bloodflow throughout the body. Imbalanced liver *chi* is reflected in the emotions as anger and frustration. Harmonious liver chi finds you calm and patient.

def•i•ni•tion

Also known as *qi* or *prana*, **chi** is your vital life force.

Spring is the perfect time to detoxify from heavy winter foods by eating watercress, asparagus, spinach, baby turnips, green onions, leeks, lettuces, new potatoes, arugula, parsley, peas, red radishes, rhubarb, strawberries, and dandelion greens. Include these foods as you transition into your spring detox program. (To go deeper into cleansing the liver, see Chapter 17 for a specific gallbladder/liver flush, plus herbs and tonics to support detoxification and healing of these vital organs.)

In the spring, it is important to begin by eating less. Eliminate fatty foods such as meats, cheese, cream, eggs, hydrogenated fats, and oils and other high-fat foods like nuts, seeds, alcohol, and junk food. Nature brings forth the young greens like dandelion, nettle, watercress, and asparagus to reduce liver excess from eating rich foods over the winter months.

Foods with a sour and bitter taste work well in liver detoxification. A drink of 1 teaspoon raw, unrefined apple cider vinegar with 1 teaspoon honey or stevia in 8 ounces of pure water several times a day provides the bitter-sour-sweet flavors needed by the liver in spring cleansing. Also fresh lemon or lime juice in water or salad dressing supported by a whole-foods diet helps eliminate liver stagnancy.

Emerging from winter, follow detox program weeks one through three (see Chapters 9 through 11) and include the liver/gallbladder flush in Chapter 17. A whole-foods diet with emphasis on bitter young greens, sour foods, mildly sweet fruits, and grains prepares the way for summer excess.

Bountiful Summer

Summer months find us active, outdoors, and on the go. Summer represents the Fire element, which rules the heart and small intestine. It is easy to overdo consumption of heavy meats and mucous-forming foods such as cheese and ice cream. Heart disease develops from eating these foods in excess. The bounty of summertime calls for excess in the variety of fruits and vegetables that cool and nourish the body.

Hot temperatures cause expansion, and sweating is one way the body cools itself while eliminating toxins. Moisture, minerals, and natural oils are also released, so drink plenty of warm or room-temperature water, use extra-virgin olive oil, and eat raw and lightly cooked vegetables to replace these nutrients. Avoid drinking cold drinks and frozen desserts, as they contract the organs, hold in heat, weaken the digestive system, and prevent you from sweating.

Bitter taste supports the Fire element. Include bitter greens, raw vegetable salads, cooling fruits, and hot peppers, which cool by bringing internal heat to the surface to be released.

Summer foods in season include apricots, blueberries, cherries, eggplant, fresh herbs, green beans, hot peppers, melon, okra, peaches, plums, sweet corn, sweet peppers, tomatoes, and zucchini.

The Watermelon Flush

Summer is watermelon time! Sweet with a cooling nature that strengthens the heart and moves the intestines, watermelon is both a fruit and a vegetable. It is a natural diuretic, beneficial for the kidneys, bladder, and stomach. Nothing quenches a summer thirst like a juicy slice of watermelon.

Take the week before to prepare for your fast by eliminating processed foods, sugar, and alcohol. Begin to reduce the amount you eat, then three days before the fast, begin eating raw fruits and vegetables during the day and steamed vegetables for dinner. Top with a dressing made with juice of 1 lemon or lime, 1 TB. extra-virgin olive oil, and 1 clove of minced garlic.

During the fast, drink nothing but distilled water and fresh watermelon juice. The skin of the watermelon is high in chlorophyll and the rind in silicon. The seeds are good for your kidneys, so juice the whole fruit.

 Healthy Tidbits

Watermelon is believed to have originated in the Kalahari Desert.

The entire process includes two days to prepare for the fast, one to three days of fasting, and one to three days to come off the fast (see Chapter 11).

Break the fast with a piece of raw organic fruit, and for lunch have a salad of freshly grated cabbage, carrot, and beet tossed with fresh lemon juice.

Midday have an 8-ounce glass of freshly squeezed vegetable juice diluted with water, and for dinner have a fresh vegetable salad with lemon juice, garlic, and extra-virgin olive oil dressing.

Cucumber Is Nature's Rejuvenator

The abundant cucumber—another cooling, sweet diuretic plant—is perfect for quelling the summer heat. This soothing vegetable is used medicinally to …

Healthy Tidbits

The digestive enzyme erepsin is found in cucumbers and helps to rid the body of intestinal tapeworms.

- Cool internal inflammation of the kidneys and bladder.
- Nourish the heart.
- Cleanse the intestines and purify the blood.
- Beautify the skin.
- Soothe sunburn.

Try a 24-hour cucumber cleanse, either having them raw sprinkled with sea salt or juicing them in a juice extractor and drinking the juice throughout the day.

Avoid buying commercial nonorganic cucumbers coated with wax. Instead, buy them from your local organic farmer or grow them in your backyard during the summer months. Eating the skin of the cucumber enhances all its benefits. When peeling a cucumber, rub the inside of the peel across your clean face and leave the residue on to work its magic. Raw grated cucumber is a great facial mask, creating soft, beautiful skin.

Late-Summer Transition

Late summer finds the Earth element governing spleen-stomach energy. It is a time of transition, preparing for the chill of autumn and the cold of winter. A short three-day fast (see Chapter 15) helps to reduce accumulated mucus from cheese and frozen desserts, and fats from animal protein and fried foods. Your body may take it upon itself to cleanse itself with an autumn head cold, unless you help out by cleansing ahead of time.

Sweet taste supports the Earth element. Include sweet vegetables such as onions, cabbage, carrots, beets, and butternut squash in your diet. Following the detox, return to eating whole foods, including more cooked grains (millet strengthens the spleen), beans, sweet potatoes, and late-summer vegetables. Refrain from using dairy and eating fried foods. Moderation is called for as your digestive system works to rebalance and harmonize itself.

Autumn Leaves

Nature pulls in upon itself, moving energy in and downward. Autumn is the Metal element, governing lung/large intestine energy. The conditions for flu or head cold come from this internal deepening as your body throws off excess mucus, toxins, and inferior oils. Foods with a sour taste help with this elimination: apple cider vinegar, lemons, limes, grapes, sauerkraut, pickles, and sourdough breads. Dairy can be in the form of goat or sheep's yogurt, but in moderation and eaten with other foods.

Pungent foods such as spices, ginger, and black pepper support the Metal element. These stimulate the appetite and help with the assimilation of food. Include pungent tastes with seasonal fall foods such as apples, grapes, broccoli, brussels sprouts, cauliflower, collards, grapes, kale, pears, persimmons, pumpkins, winter squash, and yams.

Purifying Grape Flush

Sweet and sour in flavor, the small grape is a powerful blood cleanser and intestinal broom. A one-day red-grape-juice fast or mono-food cleanse (eating only red grapes for 24 hours) has been known to restore a youthful flow to the circulatory system. High in vitamin C and diuretic properties, grapes help to reduce excess body fluids and bladder inflammation.

Take the week before to prepare for your fast by eliminating processed foods, sugar, and alcohol. Begin to reduce the amount you eat, then three days before the fast begin eating raw fruits and vegetables during the day and steamed vegetables for dinner. Top with lemon or lime juice, extra-virgin olive oil, and garlic dressing.

During the fast, drink nothing but distilled water and fresh grape juice. Use the dark-skin grapes for blood building and strengthening. The entire process includes two days to prepare for the fast, one to three days of fasting, and one to three days to come off the fast. One cup of grape juice yields 28 milligrams of calcium, 30 milligrams of phosphorus, 0.8 milligram of iron, 5 milligrams of sodium, 293 milligrams of potassium, and small amounts of vitamins A, B-complex, and C.

Break the fast with a piece of raw organic fruit, and for lunch have a salad of freshly grated cabbage, carrot, and beet tossed with fresh lemon juice.

Midday, have an 8-ounce glass of freshly squeezed vegetable juice diluted with water, and for dinner have a fresh vegetable salad with lemon juice, garlic, and extra-virgin olive oil dressing.

When buying grapes, look for plump, ripe fruit with good color and pliable green stems. America imports grapes from countries that spray crops with DDT, a known carcinogenic poison. Make sure to buy only certified, organically grown grapes and wash them well before using.

> **Pure Insights** _____
>
> According to Ayurveda [a holistic system of medicine from India], each food has a particular taste that correlates to its digestive action and that has a bearing on the balance of the elements. This taste is not a coincidence but is a direct result of the bio-chemical traits of the food and therefore also of its pharmaceutical properties. There are six tastes: sweet, sour, pungent, bitter, salty, and astringent.
>
> —Ingrid Naiman, *Taste and the Elements*

Bone-Strengthening Kale

A member of the cabbage family, kale has a warming nature with a bitter, pungent, sweet flavor. It is high in calcium and sulfur and is a rich source of chlorophyll, iron, and vitamin A. It is best picked right after the first frost, when it yields a tender, delicious, dark-green leaf. Combine kale with other autumn vegetables for a one- to three-day detox of raw and lightly cooked vegetables only.

Take the week before to prepare by eliminating processed foods, sugar, alcohol, and dairy from your diet. Three days before, begin to reduce the amount you eat. The day before your vegetable cleanse, eat raw fruits and vegetables during the day and steamed vegetables for dinner. Top with lemon or lime juice, extra-virgin olive oil, and garlic dressing. Upon rising, juice two carrots, four leaves of kale (plus stem), two stalks of celery, and a clove of garlic. Dilute with water and drink.

For lunch have a raw vegetable salad with a variety of greens, grated carrot and beet, red onion, radish, and lightly cooked kale and fresh sprouts. Top with lemon or lime juice, extra-virgin olive oil, and garlic dressing.

For dinner have a bowl of lightly steamed vegetables, including kale, collards, spinach, cabbage, carrot, bok choy, cauliflower, and Swiss chard. Top with unfiltered apple cider vinegar, extra-virgin olive oil, and garlic dressing.

Break the fast with a bowl of soft, cooked brown rice; for lunch have warm vegetable miso soup and green salad; at midday have an 8-ounce glass of freshly squeezed vegetable juice; and for dinner have cooked grain, a vegetable stir-fry with beans or fish, and fresh vegetable salad with lemon juice, garlic, and extra-virgin olive oil dressing.

This is a quick and easy detox to do when a liquid fast seems too severe or when taking medications.

Winter Blues Relief

Winter takes us deep into hibernation—staying warm, adding a few pounds, and eating heavy stews, hearty casseroles, and warming soups. The Water element governs kidney-bladder energy. The foods to eat should include salty and bitter flavors, which take the heat deeper into the body. These can include vegetable miso soup, cooked greens, burdock root, sea vegetables, barley, whole oats, and quinoa. Eating raw, cooling foods weakens the digestion and chills the body.

Seasonal winter foods include beets, cabbage, carrots, citrus fruits, daikon radishes, onions, rutabagas, turnips, and winter squash.

Brown Rice, the Great Equalizer

Winter fasting can prove cold and difficult because there's no heat in the furnace from digesting food. Rather than a liquid fast, consider doing a brown-rice fast. A mono-fast of warm cooked grains helps strengthen the spleen-pancreas, calms the stomach, rids the body of toxins, increases mental clarity, and increases energy. Brown rice, cooked with lots of water, is concentrated in B vitamins and beneficial for the nervous system. Eat three small bowls of cooked brown rice a day, or 1 teaspoon whenever you are hungry.

It is important to liquefy the rice by chewing it very well before swallowing. Do not take any other foods or drink any liquid except a few cups of Kukicha (roasted twig) tea. Drink small amounts of water if thirsty. When breaking the fast have only lightly cooked fruits, vegetables, and soupy grains.

Cooked Brown Rice

Makes about 5 cups

1 cup short-grain brown rice, rinsed

½ tsp. mineral-rich sea salt

6 cups pure water

In a medium-size slow cooker combine all ingredients and soak for 8 hours. Turn slow cooker to low and cook overnight. Rice will be soft and somewhat soupy.

Carrots for the Eyes

It is the extremely high beta carotene content that makes carrots good for your eyes and helpful for protecting your body from disease. Beta carotene is part of a group of compounds called carotenoids, found in fruits and vegetables. It is changed by your body into vitamin A, boosts the immune system, and fights against the ravages of free radicals in your system.

Healthy Tidbits

Compared with the many people who consume a dietary pattern with only small amounts of fruits and vegetables, those who eat more generous amounts as part of a healthful diet are likely to have reduced risk of chronic diseases, including stroke and perhaps other cardiovascular diseases, type 2 diabetes, and cancers in certain sites (oral cavity and pharynx, larynx, lung, esophagus, stomach, and colon-rectum). Diets rich in foods containing fiber, such as fruits, vegetables, and whole grains, may reduce the risk of coronary heart disease.

—The U.S. government's 2005 *Dietary Guidelines for Americans*

According to the U.S. Department of Agriculture, three raw carrots contain the following nutrients:

- ◆ 2 grams of protein
- ◆ 21 grams of carbohydrates
- ◆ 60 milligrams of calcium
- ◆ 1 milligram of iron

- ◆ 696 milligrams of potassium
- ◆ 60000 International Units of vitamin A
- ◆ 19 milligrams of vitamin C
- ◆ 30 microgram of folate

Carrots also have trace amounts of other vitamins and minerals, making them a rich source of nutrients and ideal for juicing. Carrot juice can be high in sugar and might be too much for people with hypoglycemia. Make sure to dilute the juice by half with distilled water. However, by juicing the carrots you are better able to absorb their phytochemicals.

Take the week before to prepare for the fast by eliminating processed food, dairy, wheat, sugar, and alcohol. Begin reducing the amount of food you eat to three small meals and two snacks.

Prepare: Days One and Two

Upon rising: The juice of ½ lemon in 8 oz. distilled water. Take a walk followed by stretching or yoga and deep-breathing exercises.

Breakfast: Bowl of soft grains or raw fruit.

Lunch: Raw vegetable salad with lemon juice, garlic, and extra-virgin olive oil dressing.

Dinner: Steamed vegetables with lemon juice, garlic, and extra-virgin olive oil dressing.

Snack: Between meals have a smoothie made with fresh vegetable juice, 1 TB. flax meal, 1 TB. flaxseed oil, and a green-foods powder.

Fast: Days Three and Four

Upon rising: The juice of ½ lemon in 8 oz. distilled water. Take a walk followed by stretching or yoga and deep-breathing exercises.

Breakfast: 8 oz. fresh carrot juice diluted with distilled water.

Snack: Cup of dandelion tea.

Lunch: 8 oz. fresh carrot juice diluted with distilled water.

Snack: Cup of herbal tea, such as dandelion, burdock, or nettle.

Dinner: 8 oz. fresh carrot juice diluted with distilled water.

End Fast: Day Five

Upon rising: The juice of ½ lemon in 8 oz. distilled water.

Breakfast: Piece of raw organic fruit in season.

Lunch: Salad of freshly grated cabbage, carrots, and beets tossed with fresh lemon juice. Lifelong fasting advocate Patricia Bragg says the cabbage, carrots, and beets help to get the bowels moving again.

Snack: 8 oz. fresh vegetable juice diluted with distilled water.

Dinner: Fresh vegetable salad with lemon juice, garlic, and extra-virgin olive oil dressing.

Return to eating organic, locally grown whole foods in season as your optimal diet plan.

The Least You Need to Know

♦ Detoxing your body should be done as one season changes to another. Enjoy foods in season when planning your detox program.

♦ You can harmonize your life by knowing the five elements of nature: Fire, Earth, Metal, Water, and Wood.

♦ Spring is the time of new growth and bitter greens that help cleanse the liver.

♦ Late summer is the time to prepare for the chill of autumn and the cold of winter.

♦ Autumn harbors the conditions for flu or head colds as the body throws off summer excess of mucus, toxins, and inferior oils.

♦ Winter fasting can prove cold and difficult because there's no heat in your digestive furnace. Instead choose a single-food fast, such as the Brown Rice Fast.

Chapter 15

The Weekend Warrior

In This Chapter

- Planning your weekend detox
- All the foods you will need
- Friday: preparation time
- Saturday: time to rejuvenate
- Sunday: relax and let go
- Monday: end the detox

As soon as you decide to make a change, take a journey, or detoxify, your mind and body begin making internal preparations. The anticipation, the planning, and then the doing flow gently toward the inevitable outcome: feeling better, looking great, and improving your health. Even when you are eating well, a weekend detox can act like a quick tune-up for your whole body. It is ideal for when you want a "pick me up and put me back on the right eating path."

In this chapter, you will learn how to use the week leading up to your weekend detox to safely detoxify your filtering organs. You will find instructions and the food suggestions you will need to make your detox program a complete success.

Before the Weekend

The first thing to do is clear your weekend of all social and work commitments. These three days are yours to relax, put your feet up, and rejuvenate your body. Nothing else is important or necessary for you to do. It may be hard to find the time because of family and work responsibilities. But ask yourself, "How often do I take a whole weekend just to improve my health and well-being?" Everybody deserves some time away from it all, and a weekend detox has just what you need.

But before you jump right into the weekend, you need to take five days to begin cleaning up your diet. If you are already eating organic, whole foods, then the elimination process should be pretty simple. By eliminating foods over the course of a week, you can easily move into the weekend fasting phase with little or no difficulty.

Healthy Tidbits _____

In the five days leading up to your weekend detox, try to take a sauna, which will help eliminate toxins through sweating; have a massage to help you relax; dry-brush your skin each day to open the pores; and have an optional before-and-after hydro-therapy colonic to remove toxic debris from your large intestine.

Detox Lead-In

Your weekend detox will begin on a Friday evening, so count back five days and begin your preparations on Monday. Be prepared to remove one food a day from your regular diet by having a whole-foods alternative ready to replace what you removed. This is what it can look like:

Monday: Eliminate all dairy products such as cheese, milk, and yogurt. Substitute nondairy nut and rice milks, rice cheese, and soy yogurt.

Tuesday: Eliminate all wheat products, such as bread, baked goods, soy sauce, and pasta. Substitute wheat-free pasta, breads, baked goods made with spelt, rice, rye, Kamut, oat, barley, quinoa, millet, amaranth, and buckwheat.

Wednesday: Eliminate all refined sugar products and artificial sweeteners, including cookies, cakes, candy, soda pop, diet soda, and ice cream. Eliminate foods containing the excitotoxins MSG and hydrolyzed vegetable protein. Substitute with these sweeteners: raw honey, maple syrup, agave syrup, rice syrup, stevia, and xylitol.

Thursday: Eliminate wine, beer, and all forms of alcohol, as well as regular and decaffeinated coffee and teas. Substitute fresh vegetable juices, herbal tea, pure water, homemade nut and seed milks, fresh lemon juice and water, herbal teas, grain coffee, and unsweetened cranberry juice.

Friday: Eliminate pasteurized fruit juice. Substitute fresh organic fruit and vegetable juice. Try having one 8-ounce glass a day.

If you are looking for a quick detox but have never detoxified before now, consider doing a slower version by following Chapters 9 through 11. This can help you avoid having Herxheimer reactions, healing crises that occur when the body is detoxifying too rapidly and toxins are being released faster than the body can eliminate them. (Refer to Chapter 8 for more information.)

> **Detox Alert**
>
> Don't be alarmed if your nose starts running, you develop a headache, you break out in a rash, or you feel too tired to get out of bed in the morning. It's all part of the detox, and these symptoms will disappear after a day or two.

If you experience any discomfort during the food elimination phase, it can be due to going off sugar, refined carbohydrates, and caffeine. The lack of many pesticides, colorings, preservatives, and flavorings can cause a reaction as well. Make sure to drink half your weight in ounces of water (4 ounces every half-hour), eat three to five quality meals a day, and get plenty of rest.

Shopping List

Decide which fast you would like to do from Chapter 11, make a list of what you will need, and then go shopping. You can include your favorite fruits and vegetables for juicing—but no bananas, and save the avocados for rubbing onto your skin.

Here's a list of items you should have on hand before your weekend gets underway:

- Organic lemons or limes
- Organic vegetables
- Distilled water
- Detox herbal teas
- Soothing music (classical or New Age)
- A gentle yoga DVD
- Natural bath products
- Candles
- Essential oils
- Natural bristle body brush
- An inspirational book

During your detox weekend, keep your mind clear of clutter and negative thinking by sitting in meditation. Take 10 minutes in the morning and 10 minutes in the evening to sit in silence and quiet your mind (see Chapter 21). It is helpful to avoid watching television or films of a violent nature. Stay away from negative people who will only disrupt the peaceful mood you are trying to create. Be selfish with your space and activities in order to get the most out of your week.

Friday: Get Ready!

From the moment you awaken on Friday, your attention should be on preparing your mind and body for the weekend. Take your time getting out of bed; stand and slowly stretch your body. Do some yoga or light exercise and take a few deep breaths, using the exhales to clear your lungs.

Head to the kitchen for a cup of warm lemon water and a light breakfast of soft brown rice, cooked greens, and toasted pumpkin seeds. Prepare the greens the day before and put the rice to cook overnight in a small slow cooker (see directions in Chapter 14). The soft grains will steady your blood sugar and ease you into the morning without a sugar crash later. The greens provide needed vitamins and minerals, while the toasted pumpkin seeds contribute protein and good fat.

Lunch and Dinner

For lunch, prepare a raw vegetable salad made with lemon, garlic, and extra-virgin olive oil dressing or try *pressing* your salad fixings first. Pressed salads are ideal for cold fall and winter months when raw salads are too cooling for your digestive system. You can purchase a salad or large pickle press online or at an Asian food market. If you don't have a press, layer the vegetables, sprinkle them with salt, place a plate on top, and add extra weight (for example, a heavy can of beans) to provide the pressure. You can use any variety of vegetables; just make sure root vegetables are sliced thin or grated.

def•i•ni•tion

Pressing raw vegetables is a form of cooking them using salt and pressure. It helps you digest the vegetables easier and gives them a wonderful texture and quality.

Following is a recipe that is delicious, pressed or not. Layer the vegetables in the order they are written for best results. The second recipe is a yummy alternative.

Dandelion Watercress Pressed Salad

Serves 2

$\frac{1}{2}$ red onion

1 medium cucumber

1 carrot

3 cups young dandelion greens (or substitute endive or romaine)

3 cups watercress

Sea salt

Wash the vegetables well. Slice the red onion and cucumber into thin half moons. Grate the carrot, chop the dandelion into bite-size pieces, and roughly cut up the watercress. In a large bowl or salad press, layer the onion, then cucumber, carrot, greens, and watercress. Between each layer lightly sprinkle some sea salt. Cover with a large plate and place a heavy jar on top. If using a press, push the stopper down and lock into place. Set aside for 15 minutes while you prepare the dressing.

Lemon Miso Dressing

Makes $\frac{1}{2}$ cup

3 TB. white miso

3 tsp. fresh lemon juice

3 TB. extra-virgin olive oil

1 TB. onion

$\frac{1}{4}$ cup water

Combine all ingredients in a blender and purée until smooth.

After 15 minutes, rinse the salad under cool water to remove the salt, then spin dry. Arrange on salad plates, drizzle with the dressing, and serve. You can use the miso dressing on steamed vegetables, so make some extra and store it in the refrigerator.

Between meals have a smoothie made with fresh vegetable juice, 1 tablespoon flax meal, 1 tablespoon flaxseed oil, and a green-food powder; or you can prepare this tasty recipe with the distinctive taste of arugula.

Spinach Arugula Salad

Serves 4

4 cups spinach leaves

2 cups arugula

1½ cups radicchio

½ cup red or white radishes, thinly sliced

For a dressing, whisk together:

Juice of 2 limes

2 TB. extra-virgin olive oil

1 clove garlic, minced

½ tsp. Umeboshi vinegar

Wash and spin the spinach, arugula, and radicchio. Arrange on individual plates and top with the radishes. Pour dressing on salad.

For your Friday night dinner, choose and steam a combination of three vegetables. Cook until lightly tender, then toss with the Lemon Miso Dressing. When putting together your combinations consider the time of year and the available foods grown by local farmers. Here are a few ideas:

- Late summer and autumn: Carrots, broccoli, and cauliflower

- Mid-summer: Zucchini, kale, and turnips

- Autumn: Brussels sprouts, green beans, and red onion

- Spring: Asparagus, dandelion, and watercress

- Autumn and winter: Red potatoes, kale, and garlic

Feel free to use fresh herbs with your vegetables. Rosemary complements potatoes, while basil complements kale and zucchini. Always include a handful of chopped fresh parsley to aid digestion and cleanse the blood.

A favorite and tasty addition is to make a quick pesto sauce using fresh ingredients. Use this on your steamed vegetables or thin with water to make a salad dressing.

Detox Pesto Sauce

Makes ½ cup

1–3 cloves garlic
2 cups loosely packed basil leaves
1 cup parsley tops
1 TB. white miso
Juice of ½ lemon
Pinch of sea salt
⅓ cup extra-virgin olive oil

In a food processor, chop the garlic well, then add the basil, parsley, miso, lemon, salt, and a tablespoon of oil. While the machine is running, slowly pour in the remaining oil. Stop from time to time to scrape down the sides. Add more oil if a thinner consistency is needed.

Healthy Tidbits

When not in the midst of a detox program, you can add ⅓ cup of walnuts when puréeing this pesto sauce and serve it with a wheat-free pasta or over salmon. Truly delicious!

Evening Activities

Friday evening after a long day of work, a warm soak in the bath will get you ready for bed. Refer to Chapter 19 for bath recipes, facial masks, and body scrubs you can make with natural ingredients from your kitchen.

Have a cup of warm herbal tea and sip it slowly. Put on some soothing music, light candles in the bathroom, and add a few drops of your favorite essential oil to the water. Take a long leisurely bath, letting yourself relax completely. Have a glass of room-temperature water to drink from if you feel overheated.

When you are done, dry off and refrain from using any moisturizer on your skin. Let the open pores breathe without covering them with any creams or oils. While your body is still warm and relaxed from the bath, get into bed, turn out the light, and surrender to sleep.

Saturday: Time to Rejuvenate

Remember, this is your weekend with nothing more to do than relax and rejuvenate. Staying in bed an extra hour is one way to pamper yourself. While there, you can do some stretching and breathing exercises. Take your time getting up, then head for the kitchen. Begin the morning with the juice of half a lemon in 8 ounces of warm or room-temperature water.

The simplest fast to do is the Master Cleanse. It requires no special equipment; you make up a pitcher of lemonade to have ready when you need it (see Chapter 11 for a recipe and details on the Master Cleanse). This lemonade cleanser will help to dispel congestion from your filtering organs—great for those of you who eat cheese and yogurt and drink milk. You can use lemons or limes, both a rich source of vitamins and minerals. Use only organic maple syrup for the essential nutrients and the sugar needed to sustain energy while fasting. The cayenne pepper is used to break up mucus and provide some warmth to the digestive system.

During the morning, relax as much as possible. Sip your lemonade, read a book, do some gentle yoga, and take 10 minutes to sit quietly in meditation. This may not be as easy as it sounds. You need to get out of the way and give your body time to recuperate from your modern lifestyle.

> **Detox Alert**
>
> It may be that by dinner time you are feeling light-headed and need something more than lemonade or vegetable juice. If that is the case, lightly steam some vegetables or have a salad of raw vegetables with lemon juice. Make sure you chew each bite to liquid. This way, you're taking care of most of the digestive work with your teeth.

In the afternoon and evening, you can retreat to your home spa for a foot soak and pedicure (see Chapter 19). Before turning in for an early night, dry-brush your skin and take a warm shower. Again refrain from using any oils or creams on your skin. However, a light moisturizer for your face would be acceptable.

Sunday: Relax and Let Go

Ah, Sunday morning, yet another reason to stay in bed relaxing. After having a glass of fresh lemonade or warm tea, do some gentle yoga and meditation. You can follow the same schedule as you had on Saturday, drinking fresh juice and taking it easy.

Sometime in the afternoon, you can break the fast with a piece of raw organic fruit in season. Take your time chewing each bite and savoring the taste. After fasting, eating again is a pleasure to be experienced.

Continue to drink your lemonade or have some fresh vegetable juice in between the fruit and dinner. For dinner, have a fresh vegetable salad or steamed vegetables with a dressing of lemon, garlic, and extra-virgin olive oil. Breaking the fast on Sunday prepares you to return to work on Monday without feeling depleted from detoxing for two days.

Before going to bed, set up some grains to cook overnight in the slow cooker. This ensures you have a warm breakfast waiting for you in the morning.

Monday: End the Detox

Just because it's Monday doesn't mean you have to leap out of bed and hit the floor running. You can work back into that pace over the next few days. In the meantime, try to hold on to the calm, peaceful mood you have created by fasting. Go easy; have your lemon juice in water, take an invigorating shower, and have a small bowl of cooked grains. The world will wait for you to catch up, so savor the moment.

You can return to eating lightly at lunch with salad, cooked vegetables, and a vegetarian protein. Plan on bringing food with you to work or eat at a restaurant that you know serves the food you will need.

For a midafternoon snack, grate an organic carrot very fine and sprinkle with fresh lemon juice. Top with some toasted pine nuts or sesame seeds. Sweet and delicious! Serve with a cup of herbal tea, such as dandelion, burdock, or nettle.

For dinner, roast some vegetables and serve with a piece of grilled fish and a side salad. Before climbing into bed, have a cup of lemon juice in warm water.

Congratulations! You made it through the weekend and back into the work week. Let the good things you did for your mind, body, and spirit inspire you to continue eating the highest-quality foods. You can see how taking a few days to pamper yourself can leave you feeling invigorated and energized.

The Least You Need to Know

◆ Clear your schedule and set aside time for yourself to prepare for your weekend detox.

◆ Take five days before the weekend to prepare your body by eliminating certain foods and substituting others.

◆ Make a list of what you will need for the weekend, then go shopping for food, candles, and bath products a few days before.

◆ Friday should focus your attention on preparing your mind and body for the weekend, clearing your calendar, and planning time at home.

◆ Saturday leaves you with nothing more to do than relax, pamper yourself, and do some stretching and breathing exercises.

◆ Sunday eases you out of the fast and into Monday's return to work with a calm, peaceful frame of mind.

Chapter 16

Gastrointestinal Flush

In This Chapter

- Suffering with bowel problems
- Grain-free detox: foods you can eat and foods you should avoid
- Hidden ingredients in foods
- Specific probiotics to take
- How to strengthen your gut

Due to advances in medical technology, Americans are living longer, but are we living longer while remaining healthy and active? The goal of many people is to move into their later years with a youthfulness that has not been seen in previous generations. You want to enjoy the wisdom of experience combined with the body of an athlete. You want to have your cake and eat it, too. Unfortunately, that cake is usually made from refined flour and sugar, the two major contributors to gastrointestinal problems. That's the bad news. The good news is you can repair the damage to your colon and live that vibrant, healthy life.

In this chapter, you will find out how to keep your colon healthy, toned, and moving with regular cleansing, dietary modifications, and exercise.

Modern-Day Bowel Distress

The large intestine is the sewage treatment plant of your body. Waste product needs to move through and out quickly so there is no backup and toxic overload. What does not get eliminated has to get handled by your overly challenged liver. When you stockpile waste inside your body, you are creating a toxic landfill, which results in indigestion, bloating, gas, hemorrhoids, and anal fissures.

You also set yourself up for the many common gastrointestinal problems that plague those who eat a diet lacking in fiber:

- Constipation
- Parasites
- Fatigue
- Weight gain
- Flatulence
- Diarrhea
- Bloating
- Eczema
- Indigestion
- Acne
- Candida albicans
- Lower back pain
- Bad breath
- Age spots
- Poor digestion
- Infertility
- Dull skin

Your digestion problems may then evolve into more serious disease issues. Following is an overview of some of the most common intestinal problems and their treatments. Make sure to discuss any alternative treatments with your medical practitioner before proceeding, especially before taking supplements not first approved by your doctor.

> **Pure Insights** _____
>
> I consider all treatment plans for disease of the colon utterly futile unless the problem of small, shrunken, infrequent stools is first resolved. The bowel transit time should range from 8–14 hours. This means healthy people should have 2–3 loose bowel movements a day.
>
> —Ali Majid, M.D.

Irritable Bowel Syndrome (IBS)

IBS is caused by an intolerance to certain foods, such as dairy and grain products. Also, foods high in fat, insoluble fiber, caffeine, coffee, carbonation, and alcohol play a role. Symptoms include abdominal pain, bloating, gas, cramping, diarrhea, and constipation. Treatments can include removing food sensitivities and taking enteric-coated *peppermint oil* capsules, probiotics, and fiber products. Check with your doctor for the presence of parasites, as they can mimic the same symptoms as IBS.

def•i•ni•tion

Peppermint oil is a safe and effective way to reduce abdominal pain and bloating in the intestines. It works by blocking the movement of calcium into muscle cells in the intestines and easing excessive muscle contractions. You can purchase peppermint oil in capsule or liquid form in most natural foods stores.

Diverticulitis

Diverticulitis is weakness in the walls of the intestines, causing small pouches of tissue to bulge outward. These can then become inflamed or infected, causing pain and distress. Tenderness near the left side of the lower abdomen is common, with more severe symptoms being fever, nausea, vomiting, and chills accompanied by bloating and constipation. Eating a low-fiber diet is thought to be the cause of diverticulitis. Cleansing the intestines, healing the intestinal walls, and eating a fiber-rich whole-foods diet is the key treatment for this disease.

Colitis

Colitis is an inflammation of the colon and rectum that includes bloody diarrhea, abdominal pain, cramping, and rectal bleeding. Other parts of the body can show symptoms, such as joint pain, mouth ulcers, eye inflammation, and skin rashes. Alternative treatments for colitis include taking probiotics, omega-3 fatty acids, aloe vera gel, and the Indian herb boswellia. The recommended diet is to strictly avoid grain, lactose, and sugar. L-glutamine has been shown to maintain the integrity of intestinal mucosa by decreasing the oxidative stress on it; therefore, it's very important with colitis patients.

Crohn's Disease

Crohn's disease is similar to colitis with inflammation of the digestive tract occurring anywhere from the mouth to the rectum. It most commonly shows up in the small and/or large intestine. Symptoms include diarrhea and abdominal pain or cramping. Individuals with Crohn's should follow a grain-, lactose-, and sugar-free diet.

Celiac Disease

Celiac disease is the inability to tolerate gluten products. These include anything made with wheat, rye, barley, oats, spelt, and Kamut. Because these foods are used in things like envelope and stamp adhesive, vitamins, and medicines, you need to be extra vigilant. Because symptoms are similar to other digestive diseases, celiac disease can be misdiagnosed. Symptoms include diarrhea, weight loss, bloating, pain, and malnutrition.

As you can see, many of the gastrointestinal diseases require the elimination of gluten-based grains from your diet. This includes bread, pasta, cereal, and most processed foods. You can replace gluten products with potato, rice, soy, amaranth, quinoa, buckwheat, millet, or bean flour instead of gluten-based flour. You will find a variety of gluten-free bread, pasta, and other products in natural foods stores, or you can order products online from special foods companies.

> **Detox Alert**
>
> Check labels to make sure the product really is "gluten free." Many corn and rice products are produced in factories that also manufacture wheat products. Gluten is used as an additive in modified food starch, preservatives, and stabilizers. Wheat and wheat products are often used as thickeners, stabilizers, and texture enhancers in foods.

Digestive diseases are a plague of the twenty-first century. Hundreds of thousands of people suffer from these debilitating problems. The irony is that all this distress can easily be prevented by eating a whole-foods diet. Include a periodic detox program with intestinal cleansing, probiotics, and enzyme-rich foods to replant the colon. The results are well worth the effort.

The Grain-Free Detox

Although most of the gastrointestinal diseases have similar symptoms, they don't all require the same eating plan. A beneficial detox program would be one that eliminates all foods suspected of causing intestinal distress. This program can be used by individuals suffering from ulcerative colitis, Crohn's disease, celiac disease, or IBS.

You will need to eliminate grain-based carbohydrates, which are all forms of sugar. These foods promote and fuel the growth of bacteria and yeast in the intestines, causing an imbalance and eventual overgrowth of these organisms. This, in turn, prevents the intestinal enzymes from working so that carbohydrates cannot be digested and nutrients cannot be absorbed. The undigested carbs sit in the intestines, creating more bacteria and yeast. By restricting certain carbohydrates, you remove what the bacteria and yeast have to feed on, reducing their population and restoring balance to the intestinal ecology.

Once the intestines are able to absorb nutrients, the immune system can strengthen and your body's health improves dramatically. Because most people are unable to digest dairy products, they are restricted for you to eat. Try this program for two weeks and see how you feel.

Foods You Can Eat

Basically you will be eating a vegetable-based diet supplemented with fruits, beans, animal protein, and quality fats. Try to stay with the percentage range for each type of food for maximum benefits.

- 55 percent of your meals from raw and cooked organic vegetables.
- 10 percent from beans and legumes.
- 10 percent from fresh fruits.
- 20 percent from organic meats, poultry, fish, and eggs.
- 5 percent high-quality fats, such as extra-virgin olive oil, unrefined coconut oil, and flaxseed oil.

Look over these creative ways to substitute foods you love for foods you can eat:

- Eggs and animal protein are acceptable for any meal.
- Almond, hazelnut, or coconut meal can be substituted for grain flour.
- Roll-ups can be made from large pieces of red leaf lettuce, cooked collard greens, or kale.
- Smoothies can be made with fresh juice or water, flax or hemp seed powder, frozen fruit, and stevia to sweeten.
- Dips can be made from puréed beans and legumes.

◆ Nuts and seeds can be eaten in moderation instead of high-calorie junk food snacks.

◆ Use ground coconut, nuts, or seeds as a breading in your fish and chicken recipes.

The oils you use should be the highest-quality extra-virgin olive oil, coconut oil, flax oil (always unheated to preserve the enzymes and nutrient value), sesame oil, and ghee (clarified butter). Eating out will be your biggest challenge. To eliminate a big discussion, order a low-carbohydrate meal without any dairy. Basically, you are asking for a dish of protein and vegetables. If you have a salad, request lemon and olive oil on the side. You need to stay in control of your food, because no one else knows what you can eat.

Foods You Should Avoid

This list of foods to be avoided includes processed foods that contain ingredients that may be grain-based. Until you have them committed to memory, make a copy of this list and take it along with you whenever you go food shopping or when you eat out in restaurants:

◆ Canned vegetables

◆ Canned fruits

◆ All starchy carbohydrates (cereal grains, flour, potatoes, yams, parsnips, chick-peas, bean sprouts, soybeans, mung beans, and fava beans)

◆ All corn and its derivatives

◆ Processed meats

◆ Breaded or canned fish

◆ Smoked or canned meat

◆ Dairy products (milk or dried milk solids, soy milk, buttermilk, acidophilus milk, processed cheeses, commercial yogurt, ice cream, and sour cream)

◆ Instant tea or coffee

◆ Beer

◆ Starches such as cornstarch and arrowroot; foods containing baking powder

◆ Chocolate

- Bouillon cubes and instant-soup bases

- Products made with refined sugar

- Food thickeners: Agar agar, carrageen, and pectin

- Ketchup

- Molasses, and corn and maple syrup (for the Master Cleanse in Chapter 11, substitute the sweetener stevia for maple syrup)

In addition, avoid medications containing sugar; but before making any changes on your own, check with your doctor to see if there are any alternatives.

Some of you may need to go further and eliminate nuts and seeds from your diet. As your intestines heal you will be able to add back foods one at a time, although returning to your original way of eating will only bring back the same problems again.

Hidden Ingredients

The difficulty in maintaining a strict diet for gastrointestinal problems, food allergies, and other health concerns is knowing what is in the foods you are eating. All bottled, packaged, and processed foods will contain some form of gluten, sugar, or corn. That includes pharmaceutical medicines, vitamins, and alcoholic beverages. Genetically modified foods may contain the DNA of a plant, such as peanut, often highlighted for its life-threatening allergenic properties.

> **Pure Insights**
>
> Beginning in 1996, bacteria, virus and other genes have been artificially inserted to the DNA of soy, corn, cottonseed and canola plants. These unlabeled genetically modified (GM) foods carry a risk of triggering life-threatening allergic reactions, and evidence collected over the past decade now suggests that they are contributing to higher allergy rates.
>
> —Institute for Responsible Technology, May 2007

Knowing where to find the hidden ingredients is certainly to your advantage. Here are a few things to watch out for:

- General Foods combines wheat with coffee beans in their Mellow Roast coffee.

- Milk sugar is used in meat, candy, baby foods, and baked goods.

- Nondairy products, such as soy cheese, often contain sodium caseinate, a milk protein.

- Lactic acid, from cultured milk, is used in numerous products and is not listed on the ingredients list.

- Binders and fillers in capsules and pills have cornstarch as a filler.

- Synthetic vitamin C comes from the corn sugar glucose.

Corn derivatives can be found in a wide, wide range of products such as toiletries, pharmaceuticals, bath and body talc, aspirin, lozenges, and ointments. Food allergies are created from foods most commonly and consistently consumed. Take a look at your diet and you will find wheat, sugar, and dairy are foods you eat on a daily basis. They are also the foods causing you so much intestinal distress. It's time to give your digestive system a break and explore some new food options.

Specific Probiotics

In 2001, a joint expert committee of the World Health Organization and the Food and Agricultural Organization of the United Nations published a report on the health properties of probiotics. Over 100 experts added to the report's findings that intestinal problems like diarrhea, inflammatory bowel disease, constipation, allergies, cancer, cardiovascular diseases, and urinary-tract infections can all be traced to a lack of proper microflora and probiotic bacteria in the intestines. This only confirmed previous research pointing to the importance of these beneficial organisms in regulating the health of the immune system.

Pure Insights

Of all the polite topics of conversation, the state of one's intestines is probably at the bottom of most people's lists. Let's face it: Irritable bowel syndrome, constipation, gas, diverticulitis and colon cancer are simply not things we like to discuss. And yet, as the old expression goes, death begins in the colon. Don't believe it? Ask any coroner. Autopsies often reveal colons that are plugged up to 80 percent with waste material.

—*Vegetarian Times,* March 1998

In Chapter 6, I explained that probiotics are microbial organisms that live in your digestive tract. There are over 400 species of these organisms working to balance your intestinal ecology. When the unfriendly bacteria dominate the colon, disease and disruption can occur.

How many probiotics should you take? Current nutritional research points out that taking a combination of microflora is more beneficial than using only a single strain for multiple bowel problems. This allows a higher potential of beneficial microflora to reach places that only one strain cannot touch.

According to a study done by the Department of Biochemistry and Food Chemistry, University of Turku, Finland, the combination of probiotic strains can show synergistic effects. For instance, the adhesion of Bifidobacterium lactis BB-12 to intestinal cells was more than doubled in the presence of Lactobacillus GG or L. bulgaricus probiotic strains. A good example of this showed how multistrain probiotics were superior in treating antibiotic-associated diarrhea in children.

When buying a multistrain probiotic, look for one with both lactobacillus and bifidobacteria strains. You want one that will survive exposure to the acid, bile, and digestive enzymes of the human gastrointestinal tract. This ensures that these organisms will adhere to your intestinal cells, allowing them to form colonies, replicate, and produce friendly bacteria for your colon.

Strengthening Your Gut

Getting your gut strong doesn't mean doing a series of abdominal crunches. That's not a bad thing to do to keep yourself strong and toned, but having a strong gut or gastrointestinal system comes from having a properly functioning colon. Doing a colon cleanse is the most effective form of detoxification for your entire body.

When you detox your colon and develop healthy lifestyle habits, you are reducing the workload on all your other major organs. These organs clean the blood that comes from your bowels—the dirtier the blood, the greater the workload. Over time, with periodic detoxing, your liver, kidneys, lungs, lymphatic system, and skin will all become healthier and stronger. Your body has the amazing ability to heal itself when provided with the proper foods and nutrients. All you have to do is eliminate problem foods and eat the highest-quality organic ingredients and let nature do the rest.

Healthy Tidbits _____

Getting enough exercise can mean 30 minutes a day of interval training, such as aerobic activity, yoga, walking, weight training, or biking. Resistance training (lifting your own or other weight) not only strengthens the muscles, it also helps prevent deterioration of the bones, which can cause osteoporosis. Strong abdominal muscles help support your back and assist with proper posture.

The Least You Need to Know

♦ Americans are living longer, but not necessarily as healthy individuals.

♦ Good health is having two or three bowel movements a day.

♦ Many gastrointestinal problems require the removal of gluten from the diet.

♦ Corn derivatives can be found in toiletries, pharmaceutical drugs, bath and body talc, aspirin, lozenges, and ointments.

♦ Food allergies are created from foods most commonly and consistently consumed.

♦ Taking a combination of microflora is more beneficial than using only a single strain for gastrointestinal problems.

Chapter 17

Gallbladder/Liver Flush

In This Chapter

◆ Benefits of the gallbladder flush

◆ What causes gallstones

◆ Your liver, gallbladder, and bile

◆ Instructions for the gallbladder flush

The most common surgery performed in North America, to the tune of half a million people, is gallbladder removal … just another side effect of eating refined and processed foods. The Standard American Diet causes gallstones to form, causing great pain and discomfort. The major foods that trigger a gallstone attack are eggs, milk, cheese, ice cream, caffeine, chocolate, and fried foods. Because allopathic medicine considers the gallbladder dispensable, it is removed from the body rather than simply flushed of its stones. Flushing is a simple procedure that leaves your gallbladder intact while washing out the sediment.

In this chapter, you will learn how important your gallbladder is for proper digestion and how to prevent its removal. You will also find instructions for detoxifying your gallbladder and liver, and the long-term benefits of this legendary method.

Conditions for Flush

Let's surmise that you've been experiencing a sharp pain in the upper quadrant of your abdomen. The pain has spread to your shoulder, your neck, and now your back. You notice how uncomfortable you feel after eating a full meal, making you hesitant to finish off that pint of triple-chocolate-chip ice cream. Your doctor diagnoses gallstones and casually mentions removing your gallbladder.

With conventional medicine you have two choices: the removal of your gallbladder with surgery or the dissolution of the stones with medication. Side effects with the medication can include nausea, pain, fever, diarrhea, and hepatic injury.

Alternative medicine recommends a change of diet that will detoxify the liver and gallbladder, followed by flushing the organs with olive oil and lemon juice. Now, that's not to say flushing stones out of your gallbladder is a cakewalk, but done properly the flush offers a holistic way to remove stones and save this important organ.

Doing a gallbladder flush will …

- Dramatically improve your digestion.

- Ease the pain in your back and shoulder area.

- Give you more energy.

- Clean the liver bile ducts.

- Help to remove parasites.

I have known people to opt for flushing their stones right away, but it can prove difficult if a large stone gets caught in the bile duct while exiting your gallbladder. The smooth approach is to take a few weeks of eating a whole-foods diet as outlined in this chapter. This will soften the stones and prepare the gallbladder for the flush. Before opting for surgery you might consider this successful treatment.

Before taking on any of the procedures outlined in this chapter, consult with an alternative medical practitioner and follow the protocol with his or her expert guidance.

How You Create Gallstones

Your gallbladder is a hollow organ, making it the ideal setting for crystallized mineral salts to form stones. Stones can be of varying sizes, the small ones easily eliminated without you even noticing. These rubbery, green formations have the appearance of sand, hard pebbles, or clay. They can stay in your gallbladder for years without you even noticing them; then one day a large stone can become lodged in the bile duct, causing gallstone colic and excruciating pain.

Gallstones are the result of a congested liver not able to detox naturally. Sediment from the liver settles in the bile and accumulates in the gallbladder, blocking the bile duct that leads to the duodenum.

Healthy Tidbits

Gallbladder issues are caused by a congested and stagnant liver. Rather than just treating the symptom (gallstones), you need to focus on the cause (liver congestion). Detoxing your liver will help keep your gallbladder free of stones.

Eating a whole-foods diet and avoiding foods high in fat is a recommended treatment for first softening gallstones before flushing them from the system. In *Healing with Whole Foods: Asian Traditions and Modern Nutrition* (see Appendix D), Paul Pitchford recommends the following 21-day plan to slowly dissolve the stones. Each day you should …

◆ Eat one or two radishes.

◆ Drink five cups of chamomile tea.

◆ Add 2½ teaspoons of fresh, cold-pressed flax oil to two meals.

After the 21 days, continue using the flaxseed 6 days a week over the next 2 months.

Along with this plan, he suggests you include foods that help to dissolve gallstones, such as pears, apples, parsnips, sea vegetables, lemons, limes, grapefruit, and the spice turmeric. According to Pitchford, this program will safely remove all sediment from your gallbladder.

The Purpose of Bile

In Chapter 4, you learned about your hard-working liver and how important it is to keep it functioning properly. One role it plays is to remove any excess bile salts and wastes passed on from the spleen. The liver then passes the bile on to the gallbladder for storage. A congested liver may not be able to remove the bile salts, leaving them to concentrate in the gallbladder and form gallstones.

Your body produces bile to do the following:

◆ Neutralize acid from the stomach

◆ Break down fats for digestion

◆ Act as a laxative for the colon

Your gallbladder is the holding organ for bile produced by the liver. Bile is used by the small intestine to digest food—particularly fatty foods. When you consume a high-fat meal such as pizza with cheese or a hamburger and french fries, your gallbladder provides the huge amount of bile needed to digest all that fat.

Without the gallbladder, there is no longer a holding space to store bile. It continuously runs out of the liver, through the hepatic ducts, into the common bile duct, and directly into the small intestine. Now, when a high-fat meal is eaten, there is not enough bile available to digest it. For some people this can result in chronic diarrhea after eating a fatty meal.

You don't have to lose your gallbladder if you eat a whole-foods diet and cut way down on eating high-fat, processed, hydrogenated foods. You can get started saving your liver and gallbladder by doing a complete detox program.

Variations on the Theme

The gallbladder flush has been successfully used by thousands of people over the years. Variations on the flush have been created by alternative health practitioners, and they basically use similar ingredients but in varying amounts. Dr. Hulda Clark's protocol is often recommended for those doing a gallbladder flush for the first time. Although most protocols use olive oil and citrus juice, Dr. Clark includes Epsom salts in her program.

Dr. Hulda Clark's Gallbladder Flush

This recipe is excerpted from Dr. Clark's book *The Cure for All Cancers* (see Appendix D). All the products can be purchased on her website: www.huldaclark.com, with some items available in natural foods stores. For her gallbladder flush, Dr. Clark suggests you first do a parasite cleanse, which is outlined in her book. Once that is completed, she recommends a kidney cleanse (see Chapter 18), and for best results having the mercury amalgams removed from your teeth. A bit extreme, you might think, but according to Dr. Clark, ultimate success is in the details.

You will need:

4 TB. Epsom salts (for laxative purposes)

½ cup light olive oil (for best results, *ozonate* the olive oil for 20 minutes, if possible, or add 2 drops of food-grade HCl—hypochlorite bleaching solution—just before drinking)

1 large or 2 small fresh organic pink grapefruit (enough for ½ cup juice)

4 to 8 capsules ornithine (an amino acid that is necessary for proper liver function; it's an important ingredient in Dr. Clark's protocol to ensure that you sleep through the night)

Large plastic straw to drink the potion

Pint jar with lid

10–20 drops black walnut tincture, any strength (used in alternative treatments to kill off parasites coming from the liver)

def•i•ni•tion

An **ozonator** is a device with an aerator at the end of its hose, which is inserted into food, oil, or water. The purpose is to sanitize and oxidize by adding a tiny amount of ozone. Ozonation quickly kills bacteria and viruses in food and beverages. You can find ozonators online or from spa equipment companies.

When you are ready to do the gallbladder flush, do the following:

- ◆ Choose a weekend or day off from work so you have the following day to rest.

- ◆ On the day of the flush, stop taking all the medications you can live without, including herbs and vitamins.

- ◆ Eat a no-fat breakfast and lunch, such as cooked cereal, fruit, fruit juice, or bread with preserves or honey (no butter or milk). This allows the bile to build up and develop pressure in the liver. Higher pressure pushes out more stones.

2 P.M.: Do not eat or drink after 2 P.M. If you break this rule you could feel quite ill later. Get your Epsom salts ready. Mix salts in 3 cups water and pour this into a jar. This makes four servings, ¾ cup each. Set the jar in the refrigerator to get ice cold (this is for convenience and taste only).

6 P.M.: Drink one serving (¾ cup) of the ice-cold Epsom salts. You may add ⅛ tsp. vitamin C powder to improve the taste. You may also drink a few mouthfuls of water afterward or rinse your mouth.

8 P.M.: Repeat by drinking another ¼-cup serving of Epsom salts. You haven't eaten since 2 o'clock, but you won't feel hungry. Get your bedtime chores done. The timing is critical for success.

9:45 P.M.: Pour ½ cup (room temperature) olive oil into the pint jar. Add the 2 drops HCl to sterilize. Wash and dry the grapefruits and squeeze by hand into the measuring cup. Remove pulp with fork. You should have at least ½ cup, but more is best (up to ¾ cup). You may use one part fresh lemon juice. Add this to the olive oil. Also add black walnut tincture. Close the jar tightly with the lid and shake hard until watery, then set aside.

Now visit the bathroom one or more times to move your bowels, even if it makes you late for your 10 o'clock drink—but don't be more than 15 minutes late. You will get fewer stones.

10 P.M.: Drink the potion you have mixed. Take four ornithine capsules with the first few sips to make sure you will sleep through the night. Take eight if you already suffer from insomnia. Drinking through a large plastic straw helps it go down easier. You may use oil and vinegar salad dressing or straight honey to chase it down between sips. Have these ready in a tablespoon on the kitchen counter. Take it all to your bedside if you want, but drink it standing up. Get it down within five minutes (15 minutes for very elderly or weak persons).

As soon as the drink is down, walk to your bed and lie down flat on your back with your head up high on the pillow. You might fail to get stones out if you don't. The sooner you lie down, the more stones you will get out, so be ready for bed ahead of time. Don't clean up the kitchen. Try to think about what is happening in the liver. Try to keep perfectly still for at least 20 minutes. You may feel a train of stones traveling along the bile ducts like marbles. There is no pain because the bile duct valves are open (thank you, Epsom salts!). Go to sleep; you may fail to get stones out if you don't.

Next morning: Upon awakening, take your third dose of Epsom salts. If you have indigestion or nausea, wait until it is gone before drinking the Epsom salts. You may go back to bed. Don't take this potion before 6 A.M.

Two hours later: Take your fourth (the last) dose of Epsom salts. You may go back to bed again.

After two more hours, you may eat. Start with fruit juice. You can start eating fruit half an hour later. One hour later, you may eat regular food, but keep it light. By supper, you should feel recovered.

Gallbladder Flush Results

Expect diarrhea in the morning. Use a flashlight to look for gallstones in the toilet with the bowel movement. Look for green because this is proof that they are genuine gallstones, not food residue. Only bile from the liver is pea green. The bowel movement sinks but gallstones float because of the cholesterol inside. Count them all roughly, whether tan or green. You will need to total 2,000 stones before the liver is clean enough to rid you of allergies or bursitis or upper back pains permanently. The first cleanse may rid you of them for a few days, but as the stones from the rear travel forward, they give you the same symptoms again. You may repeat cleanses at two-week intervals. Never cleanse when you are very ill.

Detox Alert

Sometimes the bile ducts are full of cholesterol crystals that did not form into round stones. They appear as a "chaff" floating on top of the toilet bowl water. It may be tan-colored, harboring millions of tiny white crystals. Cleansing this chaff is just as important as purging stones.

How Safe Is It?

Dr. Clark has based her opinion of safety on over 500 cases, including many persons in their 70s and 80s. None went to the hospital; none even reported pain while doing the flush. However, it can make you feel quite ill for one or two days afterward, although in every one of these cases the maintenance parasite program had been neglected. This is why the instructions direct you to complete the parasite and kidney cleanse programs first.

Seven-Day Liver Flush

If the thought of drinking all that olive oil makes you a bit queasy and uncertain about proceeding, consider taking a slower way. The ingredients of the following flush are similar and follow a seven-day protocol. This program has you eating green apples for six days prior to doing the full flush.

For days one through six, you will need:

4 Granny Smith apples

2 glasses of organic apple juice

Have the apples and juice each day while continuing to eat a whole-foods diet low in fatty foods.

One hour before bed each night, mix together:

> 2 TB. cold-pressed olive oil
>
> 2 TB. lemon or grapefruit juice, freshly squeezed
>
> 8 oz. distilled water (warm or room temperature)

Drink slowly and immediately go to bed, lying on your right side. Repeat this protocol for six days.

Healthy Tidbits

Colonics and enemas are both hydrotherapies that involve introducing water through the rectum in order to cleanse the colon. The key differences between colonics and enemas are that colonics cleanse the entire length of the large intestine and require professional assistance; enemas can be done at home, but only reach the lower section of the large intestine.

On day seven, have a colonic or give yourself an enema in the morning. The colonic will help to alleviate any uncomfortable reactions to the flush, such as cramping, nausea, headaches, and heartburn. Following the colonic, drink only the fresh apple juice and eat lightly cooked foods for the remainder of the day. Eating raw foods after a colonic can cause indigestion.

One hour before bed, mix together:

> $^{2}/_{3}$ cup cold-pressed olive oil
>
> $^{1}/_{3}$ cup lemon or grapefruit juice
>
> 8 oz. distilled water

Sip slowly; when done, go to bed and lie on your right side.

In the morning, you will have diarrhea and pass the stones. Following this, give yourself an enema or go for a colonic. This step will help to wash out any remaining toxins that have been flushed out of the gallbladder and into the intestines. Use the remainder of the day to rest and relax.

Olive Oil Lemon Flush

The basic gallbladder flush uses cold-pressed olive oil and freshly squeezed lemon juice. Take a week to prepare for the flush by eating whole grains, raw and lightly cooked vegetables, beans, and fruits. Avoid rich, fatty foods including nuts, seeds, meats, dairy, and eggs.

On the day of the flush, eat only organic Granny Smith apples and fresh apple juice, to soften the stones. The mono-fast of apples will help detoxify both your gallbladder and liver. Apples have a sweet-sour flavor, perfect for cleansing these two organs.

You will need:

> 5–6 Granny Smith apples
>
> 1 cup extra-virgin olive oil
>
> ½ cup lemon or lime juice

One option is to add ½ tsp. fresh ginger juice and 1 tsp. fresh garlic juice to the citrus juice just before drinking. The ginger helps to calm the stomach and keep the oil down, while the garlic helps to detoxify the liver.

Detox Alert

The wax coatings used on fruits and vegetables help to retain moisture, inhibit mold, prevent bruising and disease, and enhance appearance. They are made from plants, food-grade petroleum products, insects, and dairy and animal sources. They do not wash off and they are indigestible to the body. Buy organically grown apples that have not been coated with wax, or peel the skin away if the apple has been waxed.

On the day of the flush:

1. Eat only green apples, beginning with breakfast and throughout the day. Have some fresh apple juice diluted by half with distilled water.

2. Beginning one hour before bedtime, mix together the olive oil, citrus juice, and the optional garlic and ginger juice. Sip ¼ of the mixture every 15 minutes until it's gone.

3. When all the oil/citrus juice is gone, lie down on your right side and draw your right leg up toward your liver. Go to sleep; you should release the stones in your morning stools. However, don't be surprised if you are suddenly called to the bathroom during the night to move your bowels and eliminate the stones.

4. After passing the stones, give yourself a water enema to clear your lower intestine.

5. Break your fast with soft brown rice cooked overnight (1 cup short-grain brown rice to 5 cups water, with a pinch of sea salt). Use a slow cooker turned to a low setting.

You can safely flush your gallbladder every two weeks until it is cleaned of stones. Continue to follow a whole-foods diet high in fiber and nutrients and low in harmful fats and additives. Once you save your gallbladder from being removed and you successfully cleanse your liver, you won't want to go through the flush procedure again anytime soon. It's best to keep eating right and keep your body healthy.

The Least You Need to Know

- The most common surgery performed in North America is removal of the gallbladder.

- Gallstones, the result of a congested liver, are the main reason the gallbladder is removed.

- Alternative practices allow for flushing stones from the gallbladder.

- Always do a gallbladder flush under the supervision of a medical practitioner.

- Eating Granny Smith apples helps to soften gallstones.

- Olive oil, lemon, and grapefruit juice are most often used in a gallbladder flush protocol.

Chapter 18

Preventing Kidney/Bladder Problems

In This Chapter

- Preventing kidney stones and bladder infections
- Herbal supplements to support kidneys
- Herbs that help the bladder
- The kidney/bladder flush
- Ginger compress for kidneys

In Chapter 4, you read about how your kidneys can be affected by eating a poor diet. These are the organs that filter waste from your blood, such as ammonia, drugs, chemicals, urea, and toxins. The toxins are then excreted through your urine. To review, your kidneys regulate blood pressure, maintain calcium levels, balance water volume, and keep the acid concentration of your blood constant. With all that work to do, you want them strong and healthy. However, given the amounts of sugar consumed in the Standard American Diet, healthy kidneys are not always the case.

In this chapter, you will find alternative methods to detoxify your kidneys and bladder. You will learn about the problems they are prone to and how to heal them with natural remedies and organic whole foods.

Health Conditions

According to the American Kidney Fund, there are more than 20 million Americans suffering with kidney problems. These problems include the following:

◆ Urinary tract infections (UTIs)

◆ Kidney stones

◆ Kidney cancer

◆ Polycystic kidney disease (PKD)

◆ Nephrotic syndrome

◆ Genetic disorders

If any of these conditions are left untreated for too long, they can lead to chronic kidney disease (CKD). This is when permanent damage keeps the kidneys from working as well as they should. When chronic kidney disease is allowed to progress beyond the early stages, the kidneys begin to work so poorly that they are said to be failing. At this point, the only treatment options are dialysis or a kidney transplant.

The causes of kidney and bladder problems have everything to say about our modern-day culture: overuse of prescription or recreational drugs, birth control pills, aspirin, antibiotics, antacids, vaginal tampons, and diuretics. Unfortunately, it doesn't stop there—not with the added threat of heavy-metal toxicity; fecal bacteria; diabetes; and excess consumption of red meats, sugar, carbonated drinks, caffeine, pasteurized cow's milk, and alcohol. All of these things add up to a very heavy load of toxins that your filtering kidneys need to process and your bladder has to eliminate. With this knowledge, you can appreciate how important it is to detoxify your filtering organs periodically throughout the year.

Kidney Stones

Kidney stones happen to approximately 1 in 10 Americans over the course of a lifetime. Kidney stones occur most commonly in men between the ages of 30 to 50, but those as young as 20 can develop stones. Symptoms of kidney stones include sudden pain in the side, groin, genital, or abdomen; nausea; vomiting; frequent, painful urination; constipation; or diarrhea. Loss of appetite and sweating can also occur.

Kidney stones are hard masses of mineral salts, called *renal calculi*, that form in the urinary tract. When the kidney's normal pH range is disrupted, minerals can clump together and form crystals. They can be as small as a grain of sand or as large as the end of a pen; regardless of size, they are considered to be the most painful of all health problems.

def•i•ni•tion

The hard masses of mineral salts that form in the urinary tract and restrict urine flow are called **renal calculi**.

The two major contributors to kidney stone formation are:

1. Dehydration from not drinking enough water.

2. High intake of animal fat and protein in the diet.

Kidney stones can be prevented by drinking half your weight in ounces of water each day and eating foods high in B vitamins (especially B6), vitamin K (leafy green vegetables), and essential fatty acids (especially omega-3s), all of which you will be eating during the five-week detox program outlined in Chapters 9 through 13. In this way, you can easily improve the health of your kidneys and prevent stones from occurring.

Bladder Infections

While it's more often men who tend to end up with kidney stones, women have the higher rate of urinary tract infections. Bladder infections affect 1 million Americans, 90 percent of these women, and are the most common cause of women seeking medical attention. Bladder incontinence affects 13 million American adults each year.

Your urinary tract includes the kidneys, ureters, bladder, and urethra. Of these organs, infections of the bladder are the most common problem. You may have a bladder infection if you experience the following:

- A burning sensation when you urinate

- A need to urinate constantly

- The urge to urinate but being unable to go

- Leaking urine

- Urine that is cloudy, dark, or bloody

Detox Alert

A common cause of bladder infections in women is bacteria pushed into the urethra when having sex.

A woman's urethra is shorter than a man's, giving bacteria a shorter distance to reach the bladder. Another problem is that the urethra is located close to a woman's rectum, where bacteria can easily move up the urethra and enter the bladder.

Not the most pleasant experience, although not as painful as kidney stones, bladder infections can be treated holistically with herbs and tinctures.

Herbs for Kidneys

Prescriptions for Nutritional Healing, Third Edition, the nutritional reference guide for alternative health-care practitioners, describes a protocol of supplements to help control urinary tract infection and maintain healthy kidney function. Take the list along to show your doctor before starting any new protocol of supplements. It just may be that he or she will have learned something from you. The list of supplements reads as follows:

- Probiotics: Acidophilus replants friendly bacteria.
- Coenzyme A: Acts as an antioxidant and removes harmful substances from the body.
- Vitamin B6, choline, and inositol: Reduces fluid retention.
- Vitamin C with bioflavonoids: Acidifies the urine, boosts immune system, and aids healing.
- Calcium: For proper mineral balance.
- Magnesium: For water absorption.
- L-Arginine: For kidney disease.
- L-Methionine: For improved kidney circulation.
- Lecithin granules: For nephritis.
- Multienzyme complex: For proper digestion.
- Multimineral complex: Corrects mineral depletion common with kidney disease.
- Potassium: Kidney stimulant.
- Vitamin A: Heals urinary tract lining.

- Vitamin B Complex: For nephritis and overall support.

- Vitamin E: Promotes immune function.

- Zinc: An important inhibitor of crystallization and crystal growth.

With kidney problems the body retains water, creating the condition known as edema. Diuretic foods and herbs are needed, such as celery, parsley, asparagus, and watercress. Dandelion root extract supports the kidneys in secreting waste matter and is used in kidney inflammation.

Herbs for Bladder

At the first sign of a bladder infection, drink unsweetened cranberry juice diluted with water and sweetened with the herb stevia. Cranberries are used to prevent the buildup of bacteria on the walls of the bladder and help with healing inflammation. Drink it throughout the day or take cranberry capsules, but avoid commercial cranberry juice sweetened with sugar.

The herb uva ursi is a bladder infection lifesaver, as is buchu, especially when there is a burning sensation with urination. Diuretic and germicidal in nature, these herbs will help flush the bladder and destroy the bacteria causing the infection. If you are prone to getting bladder infections, keep a bottle of uva ursi capsules or extract on hand and take some at the first sign of infection.

Drink plenty of water and make some fresh celery and parsley juice to help flush the bladder. When you have a bladder infection, the following seven-day detoxifying protocol will help cleanse the bladder of infection and support the herbs you are taking. You will first need to eliminate the following stress-causing foods right away, and replace them with lightly cooked vegetables, raw salads, whole grains, and vegetarian protein.

Eliminate: All dairy products such as cheese, milk, and yogurt.

Substitute: Nondairy nut and rice milks.

Eliminate: All wheat and flour products, such as bread, baked goods, soy sauce, and pasta.

Substitute: Whole grains, spelt, rice, rye, Kamut, oat, barley, quinoa, millet, amaranth, and buckwheat.

Eliminate: All refined sugar products and artificial sweeteners, including cookies, cakes, candy, soda pop, diet soda, and ice cream, as well as foods containing the excitotoxins MSG and hydrolyzed vegetable protein.

Substitute: Sweeteners stevia and xylitol.

> **Healthy Tidbits** _____
>
> Watermelon, eaten alone, is a great flush for the kidney/bladder organs.

Eliminate: Wine, beer, and all forms of alcohol, along with regular and decaffeinated coffee and teas.

Substitute: Fresh vegetable juices, herbal tea, pure water, homemade nut and seed milks, fresh lemon and water, dandelions and marshmallow teas, and unsweetened cranberry juice.

Eliminate: Pasteurized fruit juice.

Substitute: Fresh organic fruit and vegetable juice. Try having one 8-ounce glass a day.

Catch the infection soon enough and support the healing with diet, herbs, and cranberry juice, and you should not have to take any antibiotics.

Kidney/Bladder Flush

The kidney/bladder flush is similar to the Master Cleanse outlined in Chapter 11. The lemonade recipe in Chapter 11 helps to dissolve mucus congestion and eliminate it from your kidneys, liver, and intestines. Use lemon and/or lime juice; both are a good source of vitamins and minerals. Maple syrup provides nutrients and sugar for energy, and cayenne pepper works with the citrus to break up the mucus and provide some warmth to your belly. Drink 8 ounces of the lemonade four times a day for five days while following a mostly raw, vegetarian diet for that week.

You'll do the kidney/bladder flush over the course of five days. Be sure to clear your calendar and do your food shopping beforehand.

Upon rising: Drink 8 ounces of the lemonade. Take a brisk walk followed by stretching or yoga and deep-breathing exercises.

Breakfast: Have a bowl of soft nongluten grains, steamed greens, and toasted pumpkin seeds.

Midday: Have 8 ounces of the lemonade.

Lunch: Prepare a raw-vegetable salad with lemon, garlic, and extra-virgin olive oil dressing.

Midafternoon: Drink 8 ounces of the lemonade.

Dinner: Have a piece of grilled or steamed fish; a plate of steamed vegetables with lemon, garlic, and extra-virgin olive oil dressing; and a fresh salad.

An hour after dinner: Have 8 ounces of the lemonade.

Make sure to drink plenty of water (half your weight, in ounces) and include dandelion tea throughout the day.

Ginger Compress

A ginger compress is a powerful treatment for stimulating blood flow within the kidneys and for releasing stagnated energy. It also helps loosen and dissolve stagnated toxic matter, cysts, and tumors. The ginger compress is an ancient Japanese remedy used for thousands of years to alleviate various imbalances caused by faulty diet or an unhealthy lifestyle. Its effectiveness lies in its ability to enhance and strengthen the internal organs. Ginger compresses can also be used to relieve chronic conditions such as arthritis, muscle stiffness, and pain due to injury.

A hot towel soaked in a mixture of water and ginger juice is laid across the kidneys, covered, and left in place for three minutes. The treatment is then repeated until the skin over the kidneys turns red. According to Michio Kushi, author of *Macrobiotic Home Remedies* and founder of the North American Macrobiotic Foundation, the way a ginger compress works is through the use of strong heat and the penetrating nature of ginger root. The heat of the compress dilates the blood vessels, increasing the concentration and circulation of blood to the organ, which softens mucus stagnations and fatty accumulations and helps break up mineral crystallizations. It also allows for a deeper penetration of the ginger into the kidneys.

Detox Alert

A ginger compress should never be applied to the brain area; used on babies, the very elderly, or pregnant women; applied over an inflamed appendix; or used to treat kidney cancer, unless under the supervision of an experienced holistic health counselor.

Ginger, which is similar to garlic in its ability to be absorbed by the body, will further increase circulation, open the blood vessels, and break up mucus and fat accumulation. The results of using both the strong heat and ginger causes heavy deposits to dissolve, stagnated liquids to move, and the treated tissues to be nourished with fresh blood, becoming soft and revitalized.

You will need:

> A 1-gallon enamel pot with a close-fitting lid
>
> 6 pints water
>
> ¼ cup fresh hand-grated ginger (unpeeled)
>
> Cheesecloth, cotton, or muslin sack to hold the grated ginger
>
> 2 hand towels or clean dishcloths
>
> 1 bath towel

Bring the pot of water to a boil and remove from heat. Place the grated ginger in the cotton sack and tie it shut. Squeeze the sack of ginger so the juice runs into the water. Place the sack in the pot of water, and cover with the lid. Do not add the ginger while the water is boiling (this will reduce the power of the ginger). You can save the ginger water and use it for three or four treatments.

Fold the hand or dish towel so that it is 4 to 6 inches wide. Immerse the towel in the ginger water, keeping the edges dry and making it easier to handle. When thoroughly soaked, remove, twist excess water back into the pot, and replace the lid.

The area of skin over the kidneys should be exposed and the person being treated should be lying on his or her stomach in a comfortable, relaxed position. It's best to have someone assist you in doing the treatment rather than attempting to do it alone. Place the hot towel over the kidney area and cover with the bath towel. The temperature of the hot towel should be as warm as the person being treated can stand. It should not be so hot that it burns the skin. Leave the hot towel in place for 3 minutes, then repeat the procedure until the skin becomes red, about 30 minutes.

The ginger compress is very easy, safe, and effective. It works very quickly and will afford relief to anyone suffering from discomfort and pain. It can be used on most parts of the body for any number of conditions, including back pain, constipation, ovaries, prostate, arthritis, hepatitis, cystitis, and diarrhea. It can help speed up the recovery of inflammatory conditions such as bronchitis, liver inflammation, bladder inflammation, boils, and abscesses. A ginger compress can also be helpful in dissolving hardened accumulations of fats, proteins, or minerals found in kidney stones, gall-bladder stones, breast and ovarian cysts, and uterine fibroids.

The Least You Need to Know

- According to the American Kidney Fund, there are more than 20 million Americans suffering with kidney problems.

- Kidney stones happen to approximately 1 in 10 Americans over the course of their lifetime.

- A women's urethra is shorter than a man's, giving bacteria a shorter distance to reach the bladder.

- Eating diuretic foods and herbs such as celery, parsley, asparagus, and watercress helps with edema.

- Lemonade is used in the kidney/bladder to help dissolve mucus congestion and eliminate it from your kidneys, liver, and intestines.

- A ginger compress is a powerful treatment for stimulating blood flow within the kidneys and for releasing stagnated energy.

Part 5

Mind, Body, and Spirit

The fun part to detoxing your body is the chance to pamper your body with soothing baths, stimulating facials, and calming meditation. However, you will find that there is more to detoxifying than just flushing your organs. The mind-spirit part is important for helping you ease through the stress of making dietary changes, calming any physical side effects, and keeping you on track toward making your detoxification a complete and effective experience.

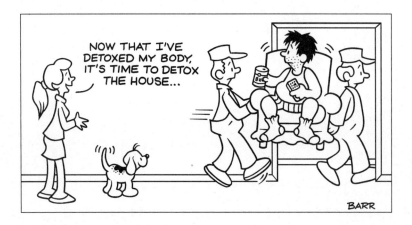

Chapter 19

Pampering Yourself Naturally

In This Chapter

- The benefits of essential oils
- Easy detox facial recipes
- Taking care of your feet
- Purifying spa baths
- Creating a home spa retreat

Complement your internal well-being by taking care of the outside of your body with natural skin treatments. Extracting toxins from the skin, removing dead skin cells, and exfoliating feet and hands leave you with a certain glow that radiates health and vitality. You don't need to buy commercial products containing synthetic ingredients when most of what you need is in your kitchen cupboard.

In this chapter, you will find recipes and instructions for facial masks, body scrubs, and foot therapies using natural food–based ingredients. You will learn how to pamper yourself during your detox in your own home spa.

Essential Oils

Essential oils are used in skin-care products, massage oils, and aromatherapy treatments and will figure prominently in the recipes found in this chapter. According to holistic practitioner Maria Prinz, essential oils are some of the oldest and most powerful therapeutic agents known to humans. Scientifically they have been documented to carry the highest levels of oxygenating molecules and minerals. They are made of oxygen and amino acids, and transport nutrients throughout the body.

Essential oils …

- Have been used medicinally to kill bacteria, fungi, and viruses.

- Lift the spirit, dispelling depressed and negative emotions.

- Can stimulate the regeneration of tissue.

- Can carry nutrients and oxygenate cells.

- Have the ability to digest chemicals.

Adding essential oils to your face masks, body scrubs, even to bath water can enhance your detox program and aid in the elimination of physical and emotional toxins. Choose the right oil for your skin type:

- Normal skin: Atlas cedarwood, geranium, jasmine, lavender, evening primrose, almond, orange, palmarosa, Roman chamomile, rose, rosewood, ylang-ylang, tea tree

- Combination skin: Geranium, rosewood, ylang-ylang

- Dry and aging skin: Almond, cedarwood, jasmine, geranium, lavender, orange, extra-virgin olive, sandalwood, rosewood, rose, vetiver, ylang-ylang, frankincense, myrrh, patchouli, sandalwood, lavender, spikenard

- Oily skin: Cedarwood, geranium, lavender, ylang-ylang, lemon, peppermint, cypress, frankincense, patchouli, Roman and German chamomile, sandalwood, juniper, coriander, lime (distilled), grapefruit, rose, rosemary, eucalyptus, myrtle, bergamot

- Sensitive skin: Roman and German chamomile, rose, palma rosa, rosewood, jasmine, spikenard, lavender, myrtle, and sage

Check Appendix D for the names of companies selling pure oils.

When buying essential oils, make sure they are the pure extracted oil and not adulterated with other oils or chemicals. Adulteration will jeopardize the integrity of the oils. They can be cut with synthetic, propylene glycol, DEP, DOP, or petrochemicals. This can be very detrimental and have no therapeutic effects when used in a treatment. Synthetically mixed oils can also produce unwanted side effects, toxicities, and allergic reactions.

Currently there are no purity standards for therapeutic-grade essential oils set by any government agency in North America. This makes it difficult to know what you are buying. When oils adulterated with synthetic ingredients fail to bring the expected benefits, consumers conclude that essential oils have no value.

A good example is the difference between pure and adulterated frankincense. Frankincense resin that is sold in Somalia costs between $30,000 and $35,000 per ton. Frankincense oil that sells for $25 per ounce or less is cheaply distilled with gum resin, alcohol, or other solvents, leaving the essential oil with harmful chemicals. A pure form of frankincense oil retails for $91.78 and wholesales for $69.75. That's a major price difference.

You can also use oils to affect your mood or improve your health in the form of *aromatherapy*. The practice of aromatherapy dates back to antiquity and is used today in a variety of alternative medical practices, for massage treatments, and in spiritual ceremonies. It is used in the treatment of depression, anxiety, insomnia, and stress, and as an aphrodisiac. The antiseptic, antiviral, antifungal, and antibacterial properties of the essential oils can be used to enhance the detoxification process.

When feeling stressed or anxious, dab some lavender oil onto your wrists, neck, and forehead to help you relax and sleep better. You can also heat lavender in an aromatherapy diffuser for the same effect. If there is a particular scent that lifts your mood, you can freshen the air in a room with this simple recipe.

def•i•ni•tion

Aromatherapy is the use of essential oils and other scented compounds made from plant material for the purpose of affecting a person's mood or improving his or her health.

You will need:

30 drops of your favorite essential oil

3 oz. distilled water

4 oz. clean, never-used spray bottle with a fine mist

Combine the oil and water in the spray bottle and cap tightly. Shake a few times, then mist the room by spraying up into the air and away from your face. Use it to spray your bed linens, and carry it with you to use in your car, office, or any space where you can comfortably introduce the scented spray.

Fabulous Facials

A good facial can be expensive, and you don't always know the quality of ingredients being used on your face. You can easily do your own facial at home using the highest-quality ingredients such as oats, apple cider vinegar, yogurt, avocado, peppermint, and even natural clay cat litter to beautify your skin.

Have some oatmeal for breakfast and save some to use later in a facial. Oats are legendary for drawing impurities out of the pores, exfoliating dead skin cells, and soothing tired or sunburned skin. Place half a cup of oatmeal in a food processor, then add some water and honey to make a paste and smooth over your face. I suggest you lay down so it doesn't slide off and on to your chest. Relax for 20 minutes, then rinse off with warm water.

For a whole-body scrub, fill an old sock with oatmeal and place it in your bathtub while the tub is filling with water. Let the oatmeal soften, then use the sock to scrub your body.

Detox Alert

Commercial facial soaps can be harsh on the skin, stripping away needed oils. Use a natural cleanser that does not contain sodium lauryl sulfate or mineral oil (a petrochemical). Extra-virgin olive oil can be used to cleanse skin and provide moisture.

Instead of using apple cider vinegar in a salad dressing, apply some to your skin. The vinegar restores the acid balance of your skin and acts as a gentle exfoliant. When your skin is peeling after a suntan or sunburn, add a cup of raw apple cider vinegar to a bath of lukewarm water. Ease yourself into the tub and let the vinegar water exfoliate the peeling skin.

Although you won't be eating yogurt during your detox, you can still use it on your face to soothe and soften skin. Try this luscious mask using yogurt and oatmeal.

You will need:

> ½ cup oatmeal (uncooked)
>
> 1 cup plain, organic yogurt
>
> Oily skin: add 1 tsp. fresh lemon juice
>
> Dry skin: add 2 TB. raw honey

Add the oatmeal to a food processor and pulse several times just to chop the oats. This makes it easier to mix and makes a smoother paste that will stay on your skin. In a medium-size bowl combine the yogurt, oatmeal, and either lemon or honey. Apply the mask to the skin and relax for 15 minutes. Rinse off with warm water.

Mashed avocado, beaten egg, honey, or other fruits such as mashed papaya or strawberries can be added to any of the facial recipes in this chapter. These foods are as beneficial for your skin as they are for your internal organs, and all without added preservatives and colorings.

Facial Mask Recipes

When preparing to do a facial mask, clear a space in your bathroom or kitchen to accommodate ingredients, bowls, and utensils. Have towels and washcloths at the ready and make sure you have a place to lay yourself down to relax. Most facial masks should stay on for 15 to 20 minutes, then should be rinsed with warm water. Begin with a gentle cleansing, then apply the mask, and after rinsing your face follow with a thin layer of moisturizer.

French clay (available at most natural food stores) is often preferred for clay-based facial masks. It is famous for its ability to draw out impurities from the skin. It is also beneficial for all skin types. Here is a recipe for drawing, tightening, and soothing tired facial skin.

You will need:

> 2 tsp. French clay
>
> 1½ TB. aloe vera gel
>
> 1 TB. witch hazel
>
> 2 drops lavender essential oil

Mix the French clay with the aloe vera gel, witch hazel, and oil. Smooth onto skin and relax until the clay dries. Use a wash cloth and warm water to remove. The mixture will keep up to four weeks in your refrigerator.

Healthy Tidbits _____

Father Kneipp, a sixteenth-century priest from the south of France, was known for his natural treatments using clay packs and poultices. He was the first to introduce clay mixed with apple cider vinegar to better draw out skin impurities.

Diane Irons, author and publisher of many beauty books, including *Ten Rules to Looking Your Best When Feeling Your Worst,* claims that natural cat litter is the same quality clay as found in expensive spa facials. Some people swear by it. If you have some (unused!) 100 percent natural clay cat litter on hand, you can try this facial.

You will need:

> **¼ cup natural clay cat litter**
>
> **Water to moisten**
>
> **A few drops of lemon essential oil**
>
> In a small bowl, stir together the cat litter with water and oil. Mix well and apply mask to face. Relax with your cat for 15 minutes, then rinse with warm water.

Clay works well for oily skin, absorbing any excess oil while extracting blackheads and dirt. Even if your skin leans to the dry side, using a clay mask can be beneficial.

Known for its pulsating effect on the skin, Indian healing clay is a good substitute for French clay in facials and can be purchased at most natural food stores or online at www.calantilles.com/Products/prod18.html. For this deep pore-cleansing treatment, you will need:

> **2 TB. Indian healing clay**
>
> **2 TB. raw apple cider vinegar**
>
> Mix equal parts clay and vinegar together to make a paste. Smooth over entire face, avoiding the area under your eyes. For delicate skin, leave on 5 to 10 minutes; for normal to oily skin, 15 to 20 minutes. Rinse with warm water.

The drawing properties of clay are not just for your face. Make large amounts of these recipes and smooth the mixture over your entire body, working up from your feet. Leave on until it dries, then rinse off with a hose or in the shower. Follow with an invigorating salt scrub and finally cover with a light body lotion.

Honey, You're Beautiful

The avocado is a natural moisturizer and can be used alone; however, combined with honey it transforms dry, pasty winter skin and brings it back to life. Honey was a popular ingredient in cosmetics during the 1800s and is making a comeback in today's natural facial products. You will find it being used in skin moisturizers, facial masks, hair conditioners, and shower gels. The consumer is demanding natural ingredients in skin care products, and honey is an effective moisturizer and healing agent.

> **Healthy Tidbits**
>
> Honey is a humectant, which means it attracts and retains water. It also acts as an anti-microbial agent, and is suitable for sensitive skin, baby care products, and treating minor abrasions and burns.

Use this facial as a transition from winter dry-heat blues into spring moist and glowing skin.

You will need:

> ½ **avocado**
>
> ¼ **cup honey**
>
> Using a fork, mash the avocado in a bowl and stir in the honey. Smooth over your face and leave on for 15 minutes. Rinse face with warm water.

Due to environmental factors, plus the aging process, your skin has a rough time retaining enough moisture and can become dry easily. This in turn causes fine lines and wrinkles to appear. It is important to keep your skin moist and hydrated. A soothing, moisturizing bath is perfect during your detox program. Fill a bathtub and add a ½ cup honey to the water along with a cup of organic milk. Relax in the water for 20 minutes and let your skin soak up the softness. While you're at it, smooth some cream and honey over your face and into wet hair for a complete softening treatment. Try to resist drinking the bath water and licking your arms. Make sure to rinse your body well afterward.

Herbal Steams

Your facial skin is exposed to the environment at all times of day and night. It is also constantly bombarded by pollutants and changing, often extreme, temperatures (see Chapter 20). As much as you try to protect your skin with creams and lotions, this exposure can take its toll. An herbal facial steam is a wonderful way to combat this harsh exposure. The steam opens your pores, expelling any dirt and pollutants. The herbs help to soothe and cleanse tired skin. Once open, the pores can better absorb beneficial moisture. This all helps to prevent fine lines and loss of skin elasticity.

You will need:

> **5–7 drops of essential oil (for an oily, acne-prone complexion, use tea tree, rose, chamomile, or lavender oil; for a normal-dry complexion, use lavender, bergamot, or patchouli oil)**
>
> **Large towel**
>
> **Skin cleanser**
>
> **Facial mask ingredients (optional)**

Bring 3 cups of water to a boil in a large saucepan. Remove from heat and add essential oil. With your face over the bowl, drape a towel over your head, tent-like. Keep your face about 12 inches above the hot water, close your eyes, and breathe in the fragrance of the oil. After about 5 minutes remove the towel and pat your skin dry. With your pores open from the steam, you can use a gentle skin wash to clean your face, then apply one of the natural mask recipes listed earlier. To close the pores when done, rinse your face with cool water and pat dry.

The herbal steam is a wonderful addition to your detox program, whether for male or female. For best effect, use it as part of your cleansing routine once a week.

Foot Care

It is truly amazing how much abuse our feet endure over a lifetime. Tight shoes, high heels, running, jumping, and dancing can stress the bones and muscles. Hot, sore, and tired is a description heard often after a long day of standing. Your feet were designed to be unconfined and bare of any covering, yet you probably go barefoot only on special occasions, such as the beach or walking through summer grass.

Detox Alert

Refrain from foot baths with salt and oils if you have an inflamed skin condition, your skin is cracked, or open sores are present.

There is nothing as wonderful for your feet as a good soaking and massage. Because all our nerves end in the soles of the feet, hands, and ears, you can massage your internal organs by massaging your feet (for more on reflexology, see Chapter 20). All the stress and tiredness melt away, leaving you feeling light on your feet once again.

Peppermint Soak

At the end of a long day, after a delicious detox meal, why not take care of your aching feet? This foot soak features peppermint oil to revitalize tired feet, and helps dispel foot odor. The Epsom salts smooth the skin, relax tired muscles, and increase circulation. The lavender will keep you resting and quiet during the treatment.

You will need:

> ½ **cup Epsom salts**
>
> **5 drops peppermint essential oil (not the extract)**
>
> **3 drops lavender essential oil**
>
> Add salt and oils to a large pan or footbath of warm water and soak for 15 minutes. When done, rinse your feet with warm water, dry, and smooth on moisturizer.

You can use other essential oils in combination to wonderful effect. In this next foot soak, the addition of smooth stones or marbles creates a natural massage that stimulates acupressure points on the soles of your feet. You get a relaxing soak and a stimulating massage all at the same time.

You will need:

> ½ **cup Epsom salts**
>
> **3–4 drops each of three essential oils, such as lemon, tea tree, lavender, peppermint, geranium, rosewood, sandlewood, or ylang-ylang**
>
> **1–2 cups smooth river stones or marbles**
>
> Pour the Epsom salts into a large pan or footbath of warm water and swirl to dissolve. Add essential oils. Place the stones or marbles in the footbath and spread them out along the bottom. Place your feet into the water and roll the stones along the soles of your feet. Soak for 15 minutes. When done, rinse your feet with warm water, dry, and smooth on moisturizer.

Nail Fungal Relief

Nail fungus is a common problem showing up in both toe- and fingernails. This particular fungus is called onychomycosis and it feeds on the keratin, which makes up the surface of your toenail. It is very contagious and lives in wet, warm places like showers, swimming pools, spas, and locker rooms. Be careful where you walk barefoot or soak your feet. You don't want to catch it, and you don't want to give it to someone else.

One of the best natural methods of dealing with toe fungus is by using tea tree oil, a natural antiseptic and fungicide that can be applied directly onto the nail. You will want to mix or top it with olive oil, otherwise it dries out the nail and surrounding skin.

> **Healthy Tidbits**
>
> When dealing with nail fungus, remember to keep your feet dry, change your socks daily, and avoid sharing towels or shoes with someone else. It is also good to keep your nails short and clear of polish.

Soaking your feet in a basin of warm water and apple cider vinegar helps to cure nail fungus. When you remove your feet from the water, shake them lightly and dry them well.

Before you resort to taking a pharmaceutical medication, try using these oil combinations for nail fungus instead. Use equal parts of each:

♦ Tea tree oil and lavender oil: Fights fungus and infection.

♦ Tea tree oil and oregano oil: Both antifungal and antiseptic.

♦ Tea tree oil and colloidal silver: Drop the silver onto the nail, let it dry, then apply the tea tree oil, let it absorb, and complete with a dab of olive oil.

♦ Colloidal silver, grapefruit seed extract, and distilled water: Shake well in a small spray bottle and spray on your nails several times a day.

Natural Exfoliants

When buying an exfoliant for your feet, look for one with natural ingredients that include any of the following: sea salt, almond meal, essential oils, sugar, seeds, herbs, and nut oils. These work to remove dead skin, smooth calluses, soothe tired muscles, and soften skin. Peppermint is a popular oil to use because of the tingling, invigorating feeling it generates. Here's a foot scrub you can make using peppermint and almond oils.

You will need:

1½ cups sea salt

⅓ cup sweet almond oil

3 drops peppermint essential oil

2 drops spearmint essential oil

Place the sea salt into a medium-size bowl. Slowly add the almond oil, stirring as you pour. Add the essential oils and mix well. Sit on the edge of the bathtub or in a chair with your feet in a large basin. Rub the mixture over your feet, scrubbing well. Make sure to get the heels and soles of feet. After a few minutes, rinse with warm water. Rub some cream on your feet and put on a soft pair of socks. Your tootsies will be feeling just fine!

The Spa Bath

If you have seen products containing Dead Sea salts, you may have wondered what exactly that means. Are they really from the Dead Sea? Authentic products containing elements from the Dead Sea can be rich with minerals, which can help detoxify your body. The Dead Sea contains over 80 minerals that can work internally or on the external parts of your body. These include:

♦ Potassium: Helps to maintain moisture and water balance in the body.

♦ Magnesium: Helps to prevent and cure skin allergies as well as tighten the skin.

♦ Sodium, chloride, and calcium: Provide mineral and water balance to the body cells.

♦ Bromine: Has a soothing effect and helps you to relax.

Healthy Tidbits

Along with skin conditions and bone and joint inflammations, stiff and tired muscles can benefit from a good soak in a mineral bath. Due to the high mineral content, regular Dead Sea salt baths can improve various chemical imbalances of the skin and body.

These minerals are present in Dead Sea waters at 10 times higher density than in any other body of water in the world.

Salts and mud from mineral-rich sources are known to heal skin problems just from adding them to your bath water. Individuals with psoriasis and eczema have found relief by soaking in mineral baths. Mineral salts are used to cure skin disorders through strengthening the skin tissues, maintaining the chemical balance of the skin, stimulating blood circulation, and eliminating toxins from the pores.

During your detox program, plan on doing a series of baths using the mineral-rich salts. This recipe makes enough for four to five bath soaks.

You will need:

> **3 cups Dead Sea salt or Epsom salt**
> **22 drops of your favorite essential oil or combination of essential oils**
> **1 TB. coconut or olive oil for moisturizing**

Mix the salt with the essential and moisturizing oils. Place in an airtight container, store in a cool dry place, and remove just enough for each bath. It will keep indefinitely.

Herbal Detox

Herbal blends are another excellent way to draw toxins out through the skin. Some combinations of herbs are used in body wraps and can actually cause a decrease in body size when used properly. If you don't want to take the time to wrap yourself in yards of herb-soaked cloth, you can pour the herbs in the bath and soak those inches away.

Here is a short list of herbs used in many herbal body soaks:

- Aloe vera: Cooling to the skin, counteracts inflammation. Antibacterial and antimicrobial.
- Mustard: Increases circulation, opens pores, stimulates sweat glands, and helps draw impurities from the skin.
- Eucalyptus: Antiseptic, balsamic, and cooling. It assists in loosening phlegm.
- Rosemary: Calms and soothes irritated nerves and muscles; an excellent antiseptic and skin tonic.
- Wintergreen: Analgesic properties help in relieving minor aches and pains. Antiseptic, stimulating, and astringent.
- Thyme: A natural antiseptic and stimulant.
- Mugwort: Used in Asian spas to ease arthritis, aches, and pains and draw toxins out through the skin.

You can tie the dried herbs in cheese cloth and hang under the faucet as your bath fills with warm water. Continue to soak the herbs in the water while you are bathing. Have some water on hand to sip so as not to become dehydrated.

Mineral Mud

Mineral mud has been found to be very efficient for a wide range of rheumatic ailments, skin rejuvenation, and detoxification purposes. It can be used as mud packs or face and body treatments. The mud absorbs large amounts of water, which gives it a considerable degree of elasticity.

Quality mineral mud is actually sediment from the bottom of the sea. The mud is an alluvial deposit containing organic animal and plant remains (algae) with a mixture of salts and minerals. The mineral composition of the mud can consist of nonsoluble tiny grains of silicates and carbonates with a high level of soluble mineral solution between the grains.

Doing a mineral mud treatment during your detox program will help to stimulate your blood circulation, maintain skin moisture, and ease aches or pains in the body. A therapeutic detox treatment would involve covering your body with heated mud for 20 to 30 minutes. The heat is slowly conducted to the joints and limbs, easing and relaxing the muscles. The mud should not be allowed to dry on the skin, but should be moistened periodically with water and rinsed off thoroughly after the treatment.

Setting Up Your Home Spa

You can easily create the atmosphere of an exclusive spa in your home with some simple tips:

- Clean your bathroom and/or kitchen before doing treatments.
- Place the herbs in a pot for an herbal steam ahead of time, then just heat the water.
- Neatly arrange towels, hand towels, and washcloths, and keep them within easy reach.
- Create the right atmosphere with aromatherapy candles and/or essential oils.
- Decide on the treatments you want to do and have all ingredients on hand.
- Play relaxing, peaceful music to set the mood.

- Keep the lights soft and soothing to the eyes.

- Adjust the room's temperature so you are comfortable, neither too hot nor too cold.

- Take your phone off the hook and turn off your cell phone.

- Let everyone know you don't want to be disturbed for the next hour or two.

Most of all, let yourself relax and enjoy the moment. You deserve to indulge your stressed and hard-working body. A therapeutic spa treatment is the perfect accompaniment to the detoxification of your internal body systems. One always complements the other.

The Least You Need to Know

- Essential oils are some of the most powerful healing agents known to humans.

- Aromatherapy is used to treat depression, anxiety, and sleep disorders.

- French and Indian healing clays are used in facial masks by all skin types.

- As a humectant, honey attracts and retains water in the skin.

- Mineral salts and mud from the Dead Sea are used to treat skin problems and rheumatic disorders.

- Creating a home spa is as easy as having all the essentials on hand and ready to use.

Chapter 20

More Than Skin Deep

In This Chapter

- ◆ How your skin functions
- ◆ The benefits of sauna and steam
- ◆ How to dry brush your skin
- ◆ Natural skin treatments
- ◆ Massage for mind, body, and spirit
- ◆ Keeping a healthy potassium balance

Weighing in at roughly 9 pounds, your skin is your largest organ. Stretched from head to foot, it covers about 22 square feet. It functions as a defense against invasion from the outside world but lets you know through the nervous system when you're under attack. The pores of your skin allow your body to breathe, to absorb nutrients and chemicals, and to eliminate toxic waste. Working with your liver, kidneys, lungs, and intestines, your skin accounts for 10 percent of eliminated waste. It is necessary to keep your pores open in order to detox pesticides, drugs, fatty foods, toxins, and environmental chemicals.

When your filtering organs are stressed from poor diet and other factors, your skin will let you know by breaking out in a rash, eczema, or acne.

Not much going on inside your body escapes being broadcast on the skin. It provides an internal report long before you even notice something might be wrong.

In this chapter, you will find age-old methods for detoxifying through the skin. You will also learn how to accelerate your detox with a special body wrap, skin treatments, and massage therapy techniques.

Sweating Through the Pores

It is a fact that if all your pores are covered you will eventually die from suffocation. In the film *Goldfinger*, James Bond returns to his room to find his paramour painted gold and very dead. She died because her body was unable to breathe or eliminate through all the very chic high-gloss paint she was wearing.

Your body secretes sebum, sweat, and salts through those pores, which allows the skin to maintain an acid mantle that inhibits bacteria from entering.

The external environment is kept at bay by a layer called keratin, interwoven proteins that literally make your skin waterproof. Keratin coupled with certain water-resistant molecules acts as a barrier to keep water inside the body while keeping foreign invaders out. Your skin, however, can also absorb certain fluids, chemicals, bacteria, and microscopic particles. Tiny lipid- and water-soluble molecules can enter through the skin and join the circulatory system.

It is this permeability of the skin that allows the introduction of herbal remedies, topical medicines, therapeutic baths, and essential oils into the bloodstream and allows toxic substances to be drawn out through the pores in the form of perspiration.

> **Healthy Tidbits**
>
> The skin is considered a third lung since it processes the exchange between the internal body and the external environment through respiration, absorption, and elimination.

In ancient and tribal cultures, there is usually a detoxification ritual utilizing high heat, steam, and hot water. The sauna, sweat lodge, steam room, hot tub, and sulfur pools exist for the express purpose of detoxifying through the skin. Although they are different in some ways, they each serve a specific purpose in healing your physical, mental, and spiritual bodies.

Benefits of Sauna

The sauna has been a primary tool of detoxification for many cultures. It is an excellent method for eliminating toxins and environmental chemicals that are stored in your fat cells. The intense dry heat of the sauna increases your heart rate and metabolism, which helps to burn fat. In this heat your circulation improves, your blood vessels become more flexible, your pores open, and you sweat. Physical exercise produces the same metabolic results, although with the muscle-strengthening capabilities.

Taking a sauna on a regular basis plays an important role in detoxifying individuals with multiple chemical sensitivity, pesticide exposure, chronic fatigue syndrome, Candida albicans, and Lyme disease. Raising the body's internal temperature is thought to kill off and/or subdue the yeast organisms and the Lyme spirochetes. Many individuals suffering with these issues report significant relief of symptoms after doing a sauna.

A complete internal detoxification coupled with the use of sauna treatments is an excellent protocol when preparing your body for pregnancy. In a 2005 study conducted by the Environmental Working Group, traces of 287 chemicals were found in the umbilical cord blood of the 10 infants studied. These included pesticides, mercury, fabric fire retardants, and stain-resistant coatings. Because these chemicals are entering the fetus from the mother, it would be beneficial for the mother to detoxify before becoming pregnant.

> **Detox Alert**
>
> Pregnant women and individuals with high blood pressure should avoid taking a sauna. As with any new health practice, consult your doctor before leaping into the heat.

Other benefits of the sauna include …

- Feelings of psychological peace and contentment.
- Feelings of physical rejuvenation.
- Symptomatic relief of minor illnesses such as colds.
- Relaxing muscle tissue after physical exertion.
- Clearing the complexion of your skin.
- Helping to relieve depression and anxiety.
- Soothing and energizing the entire body.
- Your skin becoming more sensitive to touch.

After taking a sauna, you leave feeling fantastic, as if a great weight has been lifted from your mind and body. You feel amazingly alive and revitalized, and your skin feels soft and cleansed.

The recommended length of time in the sauna varies according to your health condition. Here are a few suggestions:

◆ Sit for 15 minutes at a time in a low-temperature sauna.

◆ Sit for up to 45 minutes for a more intense detoxification.

◆ Cycle your sits by moving in and out of the sauna at one-, two-, and three-minute intervals.

Cycling in and out of the sauna will raise your heart rate, and it might be best to check your pulse or wear a heart rate monitor. For most saunas, it is essential to keep the temperature low and to stay hydrated with water and minerals. If you are sweating heavily after 10 to 15 minutes, take a break or turn down the temperature.

One way to increase circulation and mobilize chemicals from the fat tissue is to take niacin supplements for two to three weeks with daily sauna therapy.

Native American Sweat Lodge

A common belief among Native American tribes is that everyone and everything on the earth is interconnected, and each person, animal, and plant has a spirit or essence. This includes any object, such as a river or rock, and even the earth itself possesses a spirit. This belief is carried over to the tribes' healing practice of treating the whole person rather than just his or her symptoms.

Native Americans believe that illness stems from spiritual problems and that healing a person comes from restoring well-being and harmonious relationships with the community and Great Spirit or God. Disease visits those who live a negative, unhealthy lifestyle.

There are many natural healing practices involving herbal remedies, and an important technique used to cleanse and purify the body is the sweat lodge. The lodge is a dark, cavernous oval-shaped dome, representing the mother's womb. People enter through the low doorway and take their place around the fire pit in the center. The space is not large, nor the ceiling high, and people can be packed in close.

From the moment you enter the lodge and sit silently in darkness until you leave bathed in sweat, there is meaning and intent in each gesture, each sound. When everyone is seated, glowing hot rocks are brought in and placed in the fire pit, the door flap is closed, and the rituals begin. The stones used in the ceremony represent Earth as both Grandmother and Mother, an eternal matrilineal kinship. Stones are symbols of endurance in the same manner in which Earth endures. Stones absorb the power of Fire. When water is splashed on them in the lodge, the steam or vapor produced is also considered powerful and holy, the visible symbol of Creator's Breath. Such rocks or stones are sometimes called "rock people," signifying that we are related to them as we are with all creation.

Water used in sweats represents one of the two essential life-giving elements: Water and Air. Also, a talking stick (a twig or green bough from the sacred plants of willow or cedar) is often passed so that everyone has an opportunity to speak and to listen.

Through a combination of silence, singing, praying, and sharing from the heart, sweat lodges become the heart of a community. The sweat lodge experience is very holistic, with innumerable benefits to be experienced physically, mentally, and spiritually. It is seen as a microcosm of the cosmos.

People are often unclothed in the sweat lodge; and like the womb, it is a dark but secure and nurturing place. A womb does not produce a healthy fetus if contaminated with infection or impurities, and neither can a sweat lodge produce a healthy spiritual birth or renewal if penetrated with unhealthiness or impure intent such as drugs or alcohol.

Participants in a sweat rite are not unlike the fetus in a womb; both can be vulnerable to improper influences. Spiritual life deserves no less care than the physical life. A participant's sincere and positive intent is very important.

> ### Pure Insights
>
> We prefer to go into the sacred sweat lodge stripped of all our clothes, symbols, badges of education, status and wealth, camouflages or other coverings which feed the human ego. We go naked as a newborn into the womb of our Mother Earth; humble, pure, innocent and prepared for nurturing. And, in most cases we come out reborn and re-created.
>
> —Medicine Grizzly-Bear Lake, traditional Native healer

The lodge is often built (or renewed) during the morning of the chosen "Sweat Day." People fast while working on the lodge to help their intent remain focused, pure. Prayer is offered as willow or other saplings are cut, as holes are dug for the placement of saplings, and as the pit for the hot rocks is excavated. Tobacco, a powerful herb, is often used for offerings, a visible "amen" to prayer. Such lodges can be, and often are, a portal for communication with a Higher Power, the Creator; it is very necessary to exercise care and good intent in all things connected with a sweat lodge, its construction, and its rites.

Today many individuals not of Native American descent participate in the sweat lodge rituals under the guidance of a Native American spiritual guide. To find one in your area, ask about upcoming sweat lodges at a local Native American education center or at shops that carry Native American spiritual supplies.

Dry Skin Brushing

Skin brushing facilitates skin cleansing by stimulating the lymphatic system to eliminate toxins through the skin. It also improves blood circulation throughout the body and removes dead skin cells and debris that clog the pores. It is often used to break down and rid the body of *cellulite*, the lumpy, unattractive fat lying just under the skin.

def•i•ni•tion

Cellulite is the protrusion of subcutaneous fat into the dermis, creating a rippling, lumpy appearance to the skin.

Particularly during your detoxification, dry brush your skin in the morning or evening just before taking a shower. Have another brush to use in the shower with a natural milled soap.

You will need a long-handled natural bristle brush. You can find one at the health food store. If you are unable to find one, use a loofah sponge or a damp washcloth.

Begin with the soles of your feet. Using light pressure, brush in small circles from the legs toward the groin. From the palms of the hands circle toward the chest, against your back, and around your sides toward the abdomen. Finish by brushing your scalp with a natural bristle hair brush. Avoid brushing your face, breasts, and other sensitive areas.

Indulging Your Skin

Detoxifying through your skin can be helped along with body scrubs, herbal wraps, sun baths, and just by laying naked in the fresh air. Consider including one or all of these practices during your detox program. You can also indulge your skin at any time with one of these special treatments:

♦ *Seaweed Body Wrap:* This wrap is designed to detoxify the body and trim extra fat. Seaweed is applied all over the body like a mask inside a heated thermal blanket, stimulating the sweat glands in order to draw toxins out of the body. This technique works well for those who need to lose inches or for women who have problems with monthly water retention. A word of caution: this is a very powerful treatment, and is not recommended for pregnant women or other sensitive health conditions.

♦ *Sea Salt Scrub:* A sea salt scrub is reported to be the most popular body treatment at most spas. The primary purpose of a salt glow is to exfoliate your skin. It also hydrates your skin because the salt is combined with oil and usually some aromatic like lemon, lavender, or even figs. The typical salt scrub is followed by a shower and an application of body lotion, which leaves your skin feeling very soft and fragrant.

Here's a simple recipe you can do at home. All the ingredients can be found in your local natural foods store. You can adjust the amount of sea salt or essential oil to suit your taste.

2 cups sea salt
1⅓ cups warmed coconut oil
15 drops of your favorite essential oil (optional)
2 TB. honey

Combine all ingredients in an airtight container and mix well. In the shower, add a small amount to your hand or bath mitt and rub your skin to a rosy glow. Rinse off well.

Massage Treatments You Will Love

During your detox program you will want to have a massage to relax, but also to move toxins out of your body. Here are a few that are known for helping your body's organs to detoxify.

Reflexology

Reflexology is a healing art of ancient origin. Although its origins are not well documented, there are reliefs on the walls of a Sixth Dynasty Egyptian tomb (c. 2450 B.C.E.) that depict two seated men receiving massage on their hands and feet. Reflexology promotes healing by stimulating the nerves in the body and encouraging the flow of blood. In the process, reflexology not only quells the sensation of pain, but relieves the source of the pain as well.

Reflexology centers around the belief that specific areas on your feet, ears, and hands correspond to specific organs and parts of the body. By stimulating those areas through massage, reflexology assists the self-healing process.

These areas, or zones, also represent your energy body, and blockages of energy in the body are reflected through "grit" or "lumps" on the foot. As a therapist applies pressure in the form of massage, the corresponding area is stimulated and in this way removes any energetic blockages.

A typical session can last from 30 to 60 minutes. It is done clothed, either sitting or lying down. Check with the American Reflexology Certification Board (ARCB), www.arcb.net, for a qualified practitioner in your area.

Shiatsu

Shiatsu, also known as acupressure, is a finger pressure massage technique. Shiatsu massage therapy and acupuncture are founded on the Chinese meridian system. The therapist applies pressure with his or her thumbs, fingers, and palms to specific areas of the client's body that have been determined during an assessment period prior to the massage session.

The benefits of Shiatsu massage are many:

- Deep muscle and tissue relaxation
- Stress reduction and management
- Releases toxins from the body
- Dis-ease preventative
- Increased flexibility
- Improved blood circulations
- Reduces blood pressure
- Reduces mental anxieties
- Balances chi (energy)
- Calms nervousness
- Increases mental and spiritual awareness

Massage techniques like tapping, squeezing, rubbing, and applied pressure are used along the meridians to unblock energy blockages and reintroduce the optimal flow of chi (energy). At the end of a session you feel energized and centered, and have a feeling of calm and well-being … a lovely way to balance your energy. Check the American Organization for Bodywork Therapies of Asia website, www.aobta.org, to find a certified practitioner in your area.

Jin Shin Jyutsu

Jin Shin Jyutsu is an ancient holistic healing art which is gentle and noninvasive. According to its Japanese founder, Jiromurai, fear, worry, sadness, anger, and pretense are the cause of all disease. When these "attitudes," as they are called, are corrected, healing takes place and your whole body gets harmonized physically, mentally, and spiritually.

The session takes place lying prone on a massage table, fully clothed and covered with a sheet. The practitioner first "listens" to your pulse by holding both wrists. This indicates which areas of the body are weak and need balancing. Gentle touch, steady and never forceful, is applied to spots corresponding to specific areas in the body, supporting the natural flow of your body's energy.

Breath is very important in Jin Shin Jyutsu. Exhaling removes all stagnant and blocked-up energy, and inhaling after that makes us receive purified energy; this becomes one cycle. This cycle is repeated for 36 times as and when required to keep ourselves energetic and full of vitality.

Jin Shin Jyutsu works with 26 energy release points. Each point has a number, and each number has a number flow. These number flows are the many different ways the body verbalizes and expresses itself. For example, flow #3 has to do with one's understanding and ability to express feelings, to communicate. The energy then circulates to whatever depth the person needs. Jin Shin Jyutsu is, therefore, a modality that has the ability to heal deeply, at the root cause, often going back and handling emotional scars one was unaware of that have been causing physical symptoms. This is why Jin Shin Jyutsu treatments are so effective.

To find a certified practitioner in your area, check the Jin Shin Jyutsu, Inc., website, www.jinshinjyutsu.com.

Deep Tissue

Deep tissue massage is a type of massage therapy that focuses on realigning deeper layers of muscles and connective tissue. It is especially helpful for chronically tense and contracted areas such as stiff necks, low back tightness, and sore shoulders. Some of the same strokes are used as classic massage therapy, but the movement is slower and the pressure is deeper and concentrated on areas of tension and pain.

When there is chronic muscle tension or injury, there are usually bands of painful, rigid tissue in muscles, tendons, and ligaments. These can block circulation and cause pain, limited movement, and inflammation. Deep tissue massage works by physically breaking down these adhesions to relieve pain and restore normal movement.

Unlike classic massage therapy, which is used for relaxation, deep tissue massage usually focuses on a specific problem, such as:

♦ Chronic pain

♦ Limited mobility

♦ Recovery from whiplash, falls, and sports injury

♦ Carpal tunnel syndrome

♦ Postural problems

♦ Osteoarthritis pain

♦ Fibromyalgia

♦ Muscle tension or spasm

According to the August 2005 issue of *Consumer Reports* magazine, 34,000 people ranked deep tissue massage more effective in relieving osteoarthritis pain than physical therapy, exercise, prescription medications, chiropractic, acupuncture, diet, glucosamine, and over-the-counter drugs. Check the website www.nationwidemassage.com to find a deep tissue massage therapist in your area.

Potassium/Sodium Balance

The Standard American Diet contains from 3 to 7 grams per day of sodium, but only 2 grams of potassium. This is almost the exact opposite of what it should be. A desirable potassium intake per day is 6 to 9 grams from food sources.

Maintaining a dietary sodium-to-potassium ratio of at least 1:4 can protect against hypertension, crippling strokes, and premature death. Eating foods high in potassium and low in sodium, such as apricots, figs, potatoes, bananas, and tomato purée, can also help prevent kidney disease and heart problems caused by hypertension. Furthermore, a high potassium diet reduces risk of stroke and premature death even if blood pressure doesn't fall.

Potassium works synergistically with sodium in the body. However, with the typical intake of potassium versus sodium so imbalanced, researchers recommend at least five times more potassium than sodium. Because of their high salt diet, Americans have reversed this ratio by eating two times as much sodium as potassium. The problem comes from added salt being 95 percent of all dietary sodium.

Detox Alert

Kidney stones can form when potassium levels fall too low and urine citrate drops. (See Chapter 18 for more on kidney stones and keeping your kidneys healthy.)

Your body expects more potassium than sodium. Healthy kidneys regulate the potassium/sodium balance by excreting potassium. Potassium loss is also increased by excessive fluid loss from sweating, urination (diuretics), diarrhea (laxatives), or the use of aspirin and some other drugs.

The detox programs outlined in this book help to balance your potassium/sodium levels. The best treatment for maintaining potassium in the body is to increase your consumption of fruits and vegetables. A diet high in fruits and vegetables has close to 100 times more potassium than sodium. It is also important to include magnesium in your diet, from food sources and/or supplements. This allows your cells to better retain the potassium.

The Least You Need to Know

◆ When your filtering organs are stressed from poor diet and other factors, your skin will let you know by breaking out in a rash, eczema, or acne.

◆ Taking a sauna is an excellent method for eliminating toxins and environmental chemicals that are stored in your fat cells.

◆ Native Americans believe that everyone and everything on the earth is interconnected.

◆ Dry skin brushing facilitates skin cleansing by stimulating the lymphatic system to eliminate toxins.

◆ Massage techniques such as reflexology, Shiatsu, Jin Shin Jyutsu, and deep tissue massage can help move toxins out of the body and aid in relaxation.

◆ A diet high in fruits and vegetables has close to a hundred times more potassium than sodium.

Chapter 21

Your Mind-Body Connection

In This Chapter

- Spiritual awakenings
- Religion and fasting
- Detox the yoga way
- Meditation takes you deep
- Calm and focus yourself through breathing
- Your connection to the earth

There is this other side to detoxing your body that can have powerful spiritual implications. The holistic approach to healing considers the mind, body, and spirit of an individual. Spirit meaning the vital life force (chi) and one's connection to a Divine Spirit. Does this mean you will have a religious experience while detoxifying? Probably not. More than likely the initial experience of making dietary changes will keep you focused on buying and preparing unfamiliar foods.

And yet there is this moment, somewhere around the fourth week or just after fasting, when you experience a feeling of such lightness and well-being. You feel so mentally clear, so energized, as if you are connecting to something deeper. Some say it is to your true Self, others say it is how you were meant to feel in your body.

In this chapter, I will explore the spiritual side to detoxifying your body. I will introduce the holy men, women, and scriptures who have spoken to us through the ages of the importance of detoxification as a connection to ourselves and ultimately to God.

A Spiritual Purpose

In 1985, I was living near the ocean and reading the *Essene Gospels of Peace*, an ancient manuscript discovered by Edmond Bordeaux Szekely in 1928 languishing in the secret archives of the Vatican in Rome. Written in Aramaic, Szekely translated the manuscript to reveal the teachings of the Essene Brotherhood. It is acknowledged that one of their members was a young Jesus Christ of Nazareth.

I had been fasting on and off for many years already and so I became curious when reading the gospels about fasting for longer than five or seven days at a time. I felt ready to attempt the ultimate test for dedicated fasters, the 40-day fast. This is based on Jesus' wanderings in the desert for 40 days and 40 nights without food or water.

My plan was to drink fresh vegetable juices supplemented with Spirulina algae on occasion. It was summertime in Florida, too hot to eat much anyway, so it was a perfect time for fasting. I continued to work each day and ride my bicycle the 5 miles to work, take walks on the beach, and do my yoga and meditation. In fact, I was amazed at the level of my energy and the calmness of my mind.

After the fourth day, I had lost all feelings of hunger, and they did not return until the forty-fourth day of the fast. I knew then it was time to return to eating, so I chose a golden red mango, ripe and juicy, and reintroduced my body to the delights of eating once again. Something profound had happened to me during that time of fasting. I knew I had detoxified my body on a very deep level, letting go of chemicals I was sure had been trapped in my vital organs. Mind you, I am from the generation of kids who ran behind the mosquito trucks as they sprayed DDT along the streets in my neighborhood.

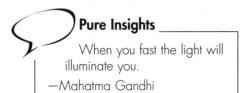

Pure Insights

When you fast the light will illuminate you.

—Mahatma Gandhi

But more than that, I came to see my place in the world in a whole new way. I came to understand that we all have a spiritual purpose to fulfill in this lifetime, and I could see mine clearly. From that experience I was able to glimpse the path I was to follow and step onto it with confidence and trust. Today I am a master yoga instructor with 25 years of experience, a nutritional counselor, a whole-foods chef, and a cooking teacher with a commitment to share my knowledge with those willing to transform their lives for the better.

A 40-day fast should not be undertaken without the supervision of a health practitioner and a clear intention as to the purpose of such a fast. I was looking to understand the spiritual significance of Jesus' denial of food and water. Although I did not place myself under the same conditions as Jesus, nor do I equate myself with this divine teacher, by fasting for 44 days I was able to shift my paradigm away from the craving for food to one of connection to the divine current that feeds us all.

Religious Food Customs

Some religious sects abstain, or are forbidden, from consuming certain foods and drinks; others restrict foods and drinks during their holy days; while still others associate dietary and food preparation practices with rituals of the faith.

The role of fasting in religious practice is seen as a sacrifice from the pleasures of food. It gives the practitioner an understanding of the suffering the poor endure and an appreciation for what one has in one's life. The body is seen as God's "temple" and fasting clears the blood of debris, which helps the mind focus on God. The discipline required for fasting is also a lesson in how to resist temptation.

In ancient times many customs sprang from a concern for the safety of food or liquids. There weren't any refrigerators or canning companies, and eating unpreserved food could prove deadly. Religious leaders of those times created rules about how animals were to be slaughtered and foods eaten. They specified days of fasting and created rituals for preparing food to ensure cleanliness and safety.

They also created rules against gluttony, excess alcohol, fooling around on your spouse, and drug consumption to better control their congregations.

Some religions believe that restricting certain foods can have a powerful impact on the health of an individual. Vegetarian diets are known to reduce heart disease and promote a longer life expectancy. The following are religions that adhere to a strict vegetarian diet.

Healthy Tidbits

In the late medieval times, one particular religion was so strict about fasting on Fridays and holy days that a man could be hanged for doing otherwise.

- ◆ Hinduism
- ◆ Many forms of Buddhism
- ◆ Jainism
- ◆ Seventh-Day Adventist Church
- ◆ Rastafari

There are some who point to the book of Genesis as proof that humans should eat a plant-based diet. "And God said: 'Behold, I have given you every herb yielding seed which is upon the face of all the earth, and every tree that has seed-yielding fruit—to you it shall be for food.'" (Genesis 1:29)

Many of our great spiritual leaders used fasting as a tool to inspire and motivate others:

- ◆ Prince Gautama became the Buddha after years of fasting and meditation led him to understand that the reason for all suffering is our human attachment to desire, outcome, and pleasure.

- ◆ Mahatma Gandhi used fasting as political motivation to move his country toward freedom in a nonviolent way.

- ◆ Mother Teresa fasted as a way to give the money she saved on food away to those in dire need. This in turn inspired others to do the same.

- ◆ Saints, prophets, and religious people have all used fasting as a sacrifice for prayers to be answered or penance for harm done in the past. By giving up that which we love so much, the food and drink that sustain our bodies, we are rewarded with the sublime knowledge that the Divine moves through each of us to work in the world.

The Yoga Detox

Probably the most thorough and profound study of detoxifying the body was documented by the sage Patanjali some 3,000 years ago and known as Ashtanga Yoga, The Eight-Limb Path. Laid out in 194 *sutras*, Patanjali reveals the steps a student must take to cleanse mind, body, and spirit:

def•i•ni•tion

Patanjali's **sutras** are guidelines in the form of a manual, which detail the path to liberation based on The Eight-Limb Path of yoga.

1. Beginning with the body, the student strives for purity through a sequence of postures (*asanas*) meant to release tensions, limitations, and a whole lot of sweat. This process removes

the impurities from blood, tissue, muscles, and cells. It also removes toxic thoughts by helping to focus the mind.

2. With the cleansing of the body, the mind awakens to an understanding of the self and the path of right action toward all species. Fasting, internal detoxification, and a vegetarian diet are undertaken.

3. A devoted student perfects each step:

   ◆ *Yama* (restraints): nonviolence, honesty, nonstealing, moderation, generosity

   ◆ *Niyama* (commitments): purity, passion, commitment, self-inquiry, and surrender to God

   ◆ *Asana* (postures)

   ◆ *Pranayama* (breath work)

   ◆ *Pratyahara* (sense withdrawal)

   ◆ *Dharana* (concentration)

   ◆ *Dhyana* (meditation)

   ◆ *Samadhi* (self-realization)

Each step is meant to cleanse the body and senses and free the mind from its afflictions of anger, jealousy, greed, pride, avarice, and hatred, bringing the practitioner to liberation and enlightenment.

Dr. Gabriel Cousens, M.D., who runs the Tree of Life Rejuvenation Center, teaches that "Spiritual Fasting is a mystical sacrifice of body and mind that opens the heart to God. It is the most powerful dietary way to become a superconductor for the Divine. Done in a full-spiritual context, it sets the preconditions for the awakening of Kundalini energy, the spiritual life force."

The benefits of doing a regular yoga practice are a strong body, flexible spine, and a clean colon, leading to a youthful appearance and long life. You become a more focused and calmer individual in all areas of your life.

See Your Way to Calm

When you have eliminated all the stimulants from your system, you will automatically feel calmer and more centered. Because your nervous system won't be jacked up on sugar and caffeine, your moods will stabilize and your blood pressure will return to normal levels. However, to help this along, you should take time for short periods of meditation.

Meditation is the practice of concentrating your mind on a single point of focus, such as the flow of your breath, a word, or an object of interest. Normally your mind is all over the place, with one thought leading to another. This prevents you from being present in each moment. A single thought lasts $\frac{1}{25}$ of a second, and in meditation you learn to let go of that thought rather than follow it into fantasy and illusion.

Following a meditation practice during your detoxification program will help to ease you through any anxious times of change and confusion. Rather than let your cravings or frustration get the better of you, sit in a quiet place, close your eyes, and focus your attention on your breath. See if you can find that moment when your exhale becomes the inhale, and again when your inhale moves into the exhale. As thoughts arise just let them go by, and come back to focusing on your breath.

Notice, also, the thoughts that keep returning to agitate your mind. Become the observer and watch the quality of those thoughts. Do you blame, judge, or condemn another? Are you angry or frustrated with your job? Rather than jump into the melee of thought, you can learn more by observing the state of your mind. Just let the thoughts pass and return to watching your breath. Refrain from making judgments or criticizing yourself; instead, repeat this simple phrase or mantra over and over aloud or in your mind to bring yourself back to calm and repose: "Om Mani Pädme Hum."

Om Mani Pädme Hum cannot really be translated into a simple phrase, although a common English version is, "The jewel within the lotus of my heart." This expression of compassion originated in Tibetan Buddhism and is based on Buddha's discovery that suffering is unnecessary: like a disease, once we really face the fact that suffering exists, we can look more deeply and discover its cause; and when we discover that the cause is dependent on certain conditions, we can explore the possibility of removing those conditions. Reciting the mantra helps to purify your mind of pride, jealousy, desire, prejudice, possessiveness, and aggression.

Healthy Tidbits

The mantra Om Mani Pädme Hum is easy to say yet quite powerful. When you say the first syllable Om it is blessed to help you achieve perfection in the practice of generosity, Ma helps perfect the practice of pure ethics, and Ni helps achieve perfection in the practice of tolerance and patience. Päd, the fourth syllable, helps to achieve perfection of perseverance, Me helps achieve perfection in the practice of concentration, and the final sixth syllable Hum helps achieve perfection in the practice of wisdom.

—Gen Rinpoche, teacher

Begin by sitting in the mornings for 5 minutes, building up to 10 minutes. Then add a 10-minute sit in the evening or just before you leave your office at work. Close the door or find a quiet place where you can sit comfortably in a chair, back straight, feet on the floor, hands resting on your thighs, and mind focused on your breath. That's all it takes.

Taking Time to Breathe

Any time you feel agitated, restless, overwhelmed, and ready to return to eating sugar-rich foods, take a moment to stop and breathe. One simple yoga exercise I recommend to my students is effective for calming your nervous system and stabilizing the mind.

Stand with your feet slightly apart and your arms by your side. On the inhale lift your arms up and bring your hands together in front of your face, but high enough that you must look up toward them. On the exhale return your arms back to your sides. Now the key here is to see if you can time the movement of the arms to match the length of the breath. At the exact moment the inhale completes, the hands come together, and at the moment the arms touch your sides, the exhale is done.

Try not to force the breath, but instead let it flow naturally while the arms lifting moves in accordance with this flow. Keep your gaze on the hands so the head moves slowly, gently with the movement of the arms. If you find yourself becoming distracted by your surroundings, you can close your eyes and focus on coordinating movement to breath.

Repeat this breath/movement exercise until you feel calm and focused once again.

Inspired to Take Action

During the course of my 44-day fast, I made sure to read only books that inspired positive thoughts. I avoided watching television, and I stayed away from negative-thinking people (not always easy to do). I remember reading a quote from Mahatma Gandhi, who said, "You must be the change you want to see in the world." There were so many changes I wanted to see happen in the world, but this simple sentence shifted something in my mind and spurred me to take action.

As you reflect in your meditation on the reality of the human condition, there is no escaping your responsibility for your immediate environment. According to health, environment, and global-warming organizations, the first thing we, as humans, have to deal with is the health of our species, which means we have to deal with the health of our planet. Are we living within nature's bounds? If we are not, then there is no way we can remain a healthy viable species, a productive responsible culture, or a compassionate people who can live in peace and harmony. To accomplish this, we must first live within the laws of nature.

To do this, we must change the technology that poisons our food and contaminates our air and water. The same technology that makes us so comfortable, that we feel we cannot live without, is seductive, addictive, and causes total pathology. Distracted by having to keep up with each day's events and stimulated by sugar, caffeine, and refined carbohydrates, our minds have become ignorant to what is going on around us.

Meanwhile, we are witness to the destruction of the human species. The evidence is there for all to see: increased cancer rate, infertility, autoimmune disease, depression, dependence on drugs, inability to communicate, disregard for the environment. According to Buddhist teachings, the major thing in your life is denial. You get up in the morning, you take care of your needs and your family's needs, and you either go to work or do what you do, as though there's nothing happening.

Yet how do you step off this destructive treadmill? Very simply, you begin with yourself. You take stock of the state of your health and then take responsibility for getting yourself better. Regardless of whether you just need to lose some weight, heal from disease, or need a physical tune-up, detoxifying your internal organs is the first and most important step you will need to take.

The *Essene Gospels of Peace*

In nature you will find the antidote to all your afflictions. As the Native Americans and our ancient ancestors believed, we are all interconnected, and nothing happens that is not felt by all beings and things of this Earth. From the *Essene Gospels of Peace* comes this understanding of our connection, our need, and our dependence on our Earth Mother: "I tell you truly, you are one with the Earthly Mother; she is in you, and you in her. Of her were you born, in her do you live, and to her shall you return again. Keep, therefore, her laws, for none can live long, neither be happy, but he who honors his Earthly Mother and does her laws."

Translated by Edmond Bordeaux Szekely, the *Essene Gospels of Peace* (www.essene.com/GospelOfPeace/) places a stark emphasis on the origin of all life. It is an inspiring text to read, once you have detoxified your mind and body, as you can better see your place in the world and understand that all life springs from our Earth Mother. With this appreciation you can take the next step toward detoxifying your immediate environment, sharing your experience with friends and family, and watching how a simple action to change can impact the world around you.

The Least You Need to Know

- ◆ Detoxing your body can have powerful spiritual implications.

- ◆ The role of fasting in religious practice was seen as a sacrifice from the pleasures of food.

- ◆ The most thorough and profound study of detoxifying the body is known as Ashtanga Yoga, The Eight-Limb Path.

- ◆ Following a meditation practice during your detoxification program will help you through any anxious times of change and confusion.

- ◆ If during the detox you feel tempted by sugar-rich foods, take a moment to stop and breathe, allowing your nervous system to calm and your mind to stabilize.

- ◆ We are all interconnected; nothing happens that is not felt by all beings and things of this Earth.

Detoxification Begins at Home

In This Chapter

- ◆ Your impact on the earth
- ◆ Detoxing your kitchen
- ◆ Just what your skin absorbs
- ◆ Living with toxic chemicals
- ◆ The energy that you use
- ◆ What makes a building sick

Every purchase you make as a consumer has an impact on the economy, health, and environment of your country and ultimately the world. We each leave a footprint on this Earth: one that can be heavy with hazardous waste or light depending on the consideration of the impact we make just living day to day. If everyone in America would make a concentrated effort to lighten their footprints, we could make progress toward preserving our natural resources and living less toxic lives.

There are so many things to think about when changing a lifetime of habits and beliefs. Clean out the inside of your body, and you're suddenly looking at your external environment as well. Once you have regained your health and are feeling good again, you won't want to return to your old way of living—and that requires a complete detoxification of your home surroundings. Really, it doesn't take much to achieve a nontoxic environment. You will need to replace certain house-cleaning products, restock your linen closet with organic fabrics, and make it a policy to recycle certain items. Once you know about the chemicals coming into your home, you will be able to do damage control, bringing order to your immediate environment.

In this chapter, you will find information on creating as healthy a lifestyle as possible in today's toxic world. From setting up your kitchen and buying food and water filters to finding eco-friendly household cleaners and air purifiers, this chapter will be your guide. Living clean doesn't mean having to be perfect. Making changes one at a time will eventually give you a healthy home environment.

If you would like to learn more about specific products mentioned in this chapter, see the books and websites listed in Appendix D for a quick referral.

Living the Clean Life

Getting to this chapter means you have looked through the rest of the book, have possibly answered the questionnaires in Chapter 1, and have set aside time to do the five-week detox program, or better still, you completed the program and want to learn more. In which case, now you are here and I have a few questions for you:

- Have you added more organic foods to your diet?
- Are you eating more fresh fruits and vegetables?
- Are you drinking half your weight in ounces of water each day?
- Are you preparing your meals at home more often?
- Are you taking your lunch to work or when you travel?
- Are you buying from the organic farmers in your area?
- Are you taking digestive enzymes?
- Are you taking a multistrain probiotic?
- Do you include a fiber drink in your meal plan?
- Did you answer the questionnaires in Chapter 1 after doing your detox?
- Have any of your symptoms eased up or disappeared after doing the detox programs in this book?

It's good to check in with yourself from time to time and ask questions about your progress. Once you have detoxified, it is important to remain focused on achieving optimal health, and having a plan of action serves as a guide. Small changes each month can have you environmentally sustainable within a year. Your plan can look something like this:

Months 1–3: Your Kitchen

Replace food in kitchen with organic, whole foods.

Replace cooking utensils and cookware.

Switch to nontoxic cleansers.

Safely dispose of toxic cleansers.

Install a water filter.

Months 4–6: Your Body

Replace formaldehyde-treated linens with organic.

Replace dry cleaning with laundering.

Replace commercial wash detergents with eco-products.

Replace skin care products with natural, organic products.

Avoid using "disposable" products of all kinds.

Months 7–9: Your Home

Replace toxic carpets with renewable wood or bamboo.

Dispose of toxic pesticides for natural repellents.

Purchase an air purifier.

Replace pressboard furniture with renewable wood pieces.

Use alternative building materials for renovation projects.

Use low VOC paints in place of toxic brands.

Months 10–12: Your Energy Use

Drive your car less and walk, ride a bike, or share rides.

Keep your car tuned or buy a hybrid.

Insulate your home to cut down on energy use.

Replace incandescent bulbs with compact fluorescent bulbs.

Over the course of a year, you can make a dramatic difference in the quality of your health, your home environment, and the impact your actions have on the earth. The eco-green movement in America has spawned creative alternative ways to replace standard toxic products with safe and renewable ones. Once you know the situation, you will better understand the need for change. Let's take a closer look at changes you can make in each of these areas.

Your Kitchen

The cookware and utensils you use to prepare food are just as important as the ingredients. For many of you, Teflon-coated pans have made cooking and cleanup easy. And though a few nicks and scratches have appeared on the surface, you never gave it much thought.

According to tests commissioned by the Environmental Working Group (EWG), Teflon will break apart and emit toxic carcinogenic particles and gas during the cooking process. Ammonium perfluorooctanoic acid (C8), the active ingredient in Teflon, has been linked to cancer and organ damage in laboratory animals. Teflon is used as a stain guard for carpets, in pizza boxes, in nonstick pans, and in microwave-popcorn bags. Consequently, it is found in the blood of 95 percent of Americans.

Pure Insights

DuPont studies show that Teflon off-gases toxic particulates at 464°F. At 680°F Teflon pans release at least six toxic gases, including two carcinogens, two global pollutants, and MFA, a chemical lethal to humans at low doses. At temperatures that DuPont scientists claim are reached on stovetop drip pans (1000°F), nonstick coatings break down to a chemical warfare agent known as PFIB, and a chemical analog of the WWII nerve gas phosgene.

—Environmental Working Group (EWG)

A simple solution for preventing your food from sticking is to rub the bottom of your skillet with coarse salt and shake off any excess. Proceed as usual with little or no food sticking to your pan.

When replacing your cookware, consider these safe alternatives:

◆ Cast iron not only provides a small amount of iron to your diet, but has excellent heat distribution and lasts forever.

- Ceramic over cast iron, my personal favorite, provides excellent heat distribution for slow, long simmering of soups, grains, and stews. Buy cookware without the nonstick coating and use for many years to come. Iron cookware keeps your arms strong lifting them around the kitchen.

- Stainless steel is actually made from a combination of metals including nickel, chromium, and molybdenum. It is safe to use, but traces can enter the food if the cookware is pitted or banged up.

- Kiln-fired ceramic and clay pots are known to improve the flavors of food. They are safe to use, but check that glazes are lead-free when buying imported brands.

The cooking utensils should be made from a renewable source such as bamboo or wood. Bamboo is an excellent material for cooking utensils and cutting boards, as it is harder than oak and a renewable resource as well. Plastic can leach into food when exposed to high heat. This includes bowls and dishes used in microwave cooking.

Store your food in glass containers and use the plastic ones to keep miscellaneous items like nails and screws, receipts, and recipes. Just keep them away from your food and out of the landfill.

Healthy Tidbits

Use your microwave to disinfect your wet sponges. Researchers at the University of Florida zapped sponges soaked in water containing E. coli and viruses. After two minutes on high, it killed more than 99 percent of the bacteria. Make sure the sponge is wet to avoid setting your kitchen on fire.

If you are going to eat the highest-quality food, you want to prepare it in the highest-quality cookware. The best only costs twice as much and lasts three times longer. It's worth the investment in terms of your health and the health of the planet.

Eating Organically

Make eating the best-quality foods a priority for yourself and your family. List it as the number-one most important thing you can do each day, and it will reflect in your health and vitality. The best lifestyle plan is outlined in Chapter 9 and gets you started on the path. Stay away from the foods that weaken your digestive system, liver, kidneys, and lungs: refined sugar, wheat flour, pasteurized dairy, caffeine, soda, alcohol, and drugs. Keep those bad boys out of your diet, and your life will change dramatically for the better.

If it seems daunting to try cooking with foods you've never heard of before, then take a few natural foods cooking classes. This gives you a chance to explore new tastes and recipes you may never have tried. Look for a class that will introduce you to setting up your kitchen, shopping for whole foods, chopping techniques, and organic ingredients.

If getting around a health-food store seems like navigating a foreign country, then call the store and request a guided tour. Bring along your shopping list and spend some time walking the aisles familiarizing yourself with the products. Read product labels as if your life depended on it, because it does. Just because it is called a "health-food" store does not mean that everything there is healthy for you. Sugar is still a favorite additive no matter where you shop. Many conventional supermarkets now carry organic products and some produce. Don't be shy about asking the manager to order products you need to stay healthy.

Household Cleaners

Warning labels on your household cleaners should be one indication that they are very dangerous to your health. They can cause irritation to eyes and skin, and inhaling the fumes can affect your lungs. Safe alternatives can be as simple as the following:

Detox Alert

When getting rid of household cleaners, check with your town or city to learn about restrictions and proper disposal of all hazardous products.

- Baking soda
- White vinegar
- Lemon juice
- Borax
- Liquid soap made from natural sources

Nontoxic cleaners are also available from reputable companies committed to keeping the planet healthy. When you spray these cleaners near your food, you can rest assured that you will be safe from any poisonous chemicals. On the other hand, your standard all-purpose cleaners contain toxic substances like chlorinated phosphates, complex phosphates, dry bleach, kerosene, petroleum-based surfactants, sodium bromide, glycol ether, Stoddard solvent, EDTA, and naphtha.

Water Filters

Drinking half your weight in ounces of water each day, plus cooking with water, equals a whole lot of water consumed by one person in a day. In 2004, Americans consumed nearly 7 billion gallons of bottled water, much of it stored in plastic. The problem here is the poor quality water in our cities containing fluoride, chlorine, traces of arsenic, lead, aluminum, and pharmaceutical drugs. Buying bottled water is not the answer either. Plastic water bottles leach phthalates, a petrochemical known to disrupt your reproductive system.

The cost to our health, our clogged landfills, plus manufacturing and transportation costs is enormous and only getting worse. What can you do about it? For one thing, you can use glass for carrying water and install a water filtration system on your kitchen sink or on sinks in your whole house.

Your Body

What you put on the outside of your body can influence your health on the inside. Sixty percent of everything you put on our skin is absorbed into your bloodstream. Not convinced? Try this experiment: slice a clove of garlic and rub it on the soft sole of your foot. Within 15 minutes you should be able to taste the garlic in your mouth—that's how fast it can move through your bloodstream.

With that in mind, consider all the fabrics, skin-care lotions, and detergents you and your children come into contact with each day. You might be surprised at the level of chemicals you could be absorbing.

The Fabrics You Wear

The U.S. Environmental Protection Agency (EPA) classifies pesticides in terms of danger to our health. Category 1 pesticides are the most dangerous category of these chemicals and known carcinogens. Unbeknownst to you, they are sprayed on the cotton crops that produced the T-shirt you're now wearing. They can easily be absorbed by your skin, as can the chemicals used in color dyes, the flame retardants in your bedding, and permanent-press shirts.

Today there are enough organic apparel companies designing attractive organic clothes, bed linens, and even workout clothes to keep you looking very stylish. Fabric dyes are made from vegetable sources and a fabric alternative to cotton is *Cannabis*

Detox Alert _____

A fire-resistant chemical used on children's clothes is polybrominated diphenyl ether (PBDE), linked to brain and thyroid development problems.

sativa L. (Cannabaceae), better known as hemp. Industrial hemp is a renewable resource. Its fibers are harvested for hemp clothing and its seeds for hemp oil. A short growth cycle of 100 to 120 days produces an economical and sustainable crop. Industrial hemp and marijuana are separate breeds of Cannabis sativa and should not be confused with each other.

Dry Cleaning

Dry cleaning your clothes can be hazardous to your health. Perchloroethylene, a known carcinogen, has been shown to cause liver, kidney, and central nervous system damage to employees exposed at work. Dry cleaning involves immersing or spot-treating a garment with "perc" as the primary solvent and can be absorbed through the skin of the wearer.

If you have to dry clean your clothes, bring them home afterward and take them out of the plastic. Hang them where they can air out for 24 to 48 hours before putting them against your skin. Better still, find a green dry cleaner in your area or hand-launder your delicate fabrics.

Eco-Detergents

Commercial detergent products are specially designed to clean synthetic fabrics and are derived from petrochemicals and phosphates … an environmental nightmare, as all that detergent ends up in our streams and waterways upsetting the balance of nature. They cause blooms of algae to take over and deplete the dissolved oxygen fish need to live. Some detergent may even contain naphthalene or phenol, both hazardous substances. People sensitive to these compounds may find it hard to tolerate detergents or the fragrances they are scented with.

A few natural products you have in the house can work wonders in your laundry:

- To keep colors bright, add a cup of white vinegar to the wash (to avoid toxic fumes, *do not* use with bleach).

- One half to three quarters of a cup of baking soda will leave clothes soft and fresh smelling.

- Silks and wools may be hand-washed with mild soap or a protein shampoo.

- Items containing down or feathers can be washed with a mild soap or baking soda.

Eco-friendly detergents have been available for some time in the marketplace. They are biodegradable and very effective without the use of phosphates, chemicals, and fragrances. They work well with cotton, hemp, synthetic fabrics, and blends, including most no-iron fabrics.

Personal-Care Products

Personal-care products encompass everything from bath gels, body lotions, makeup, sunscreen, hair dye, antiperspirants, soaps, toothpaste, mouthwash, and shampoos. A good adage to live by is "if you won't eat it, then don't put it on your skin." The products you may be presently using are created from over 3,000 ingredients, many harmful to your health. Parabens, urea, propylene glycol, sodium, lauryl sulfate, PEGs, and petrochemicals are but a few. Most of them have been tested on animals under conditions you would not want to subject your pets to.

Look for products made with natural ingredients, preferably organic. You might be surprised to find that these body-friendly skin-care products are more effective in treating your skin, hair, and mouth than the chemical-based products. Many natural products are fragrance-free or use essential oils. Oftentimes a store will have a sample of the product you can smell before buying. It's a good way to know if your can live with it day after day.

Disposables

How many times a day do you use an item and then throw it away? Americans have become a disposable culture. A cup of coffee to go, then toss it in the garbage when done. Endless numbers of grocery bags, light, cheap, durable, and used by the trillions, end up in the landfill, along roadways, and floating in rivers and lakes, harming wildlife and trashing nature. Disposable razors, batteries, chopsticks, utensils, paper goods, food packaging, cleaning supplies … the list goes on. All these items load up our landfills or go up in smoke from your local garbage incinerator, ending up in our lungs.

Take a look at the recyclable products or disposables that break down in a short period of time. Recharge your batteries, own a razor that will last a long time, bring your own cup when buying coffee, and recycle your plastics and paper properly.

Your Home

Let's take a look at what's floating around inside your home. It's called off-gassing and comes from new items such as carpets, furniture, paint, drywall, and others that emit toxic and hazardous fumes. The number-one bad guy used in all these products is formaldehyde, and it is inhaled in every home to some degree. The concentrations can vary depending on your home's age and the items you purchase, but be assured it can cause some very serious health problems. As a matter of fact, the Environmental Defense Scoreboard has ranked formaldehyde at the top of the list for most hazardous chemical to human health and ecosystems.

Carpets and Furniture

Carpets and new furniture are primary items that emit formaldehyde, along with toluene, xylene, and benzene. These toxic chemicals can be found in the fiber-bonding material, dyes, backing glues, fire retardants, latex binder, fungicides, and antistatic and stain-resistant treatments. The good news is you can purchase a nontoxic carpet made from natural fibers such as wool, jute, sisal, sea grass, coir, or recycled PET (polyester) plastic.

Detox Alert

Off-gassing from new carpets can persist at high levels for up to three years after installation. There are as many as 120 chemicals in a typical sample of carpet. In general, the most active stage of off-gassing is from one to three months.

Many of the chemicals in your furniture, including formaldehyde, come from the pressboard used to replace solid wood. Also, new furniture fabric is treated with stain-resistant chemicals, giving you a double dose of fumes. Renewable, nontoxic furniture is available and just as stylish as anything you can find in the commercial market. Go online to find companies that make carpets and furniture with an eye toward keeping you healthy while preserving the earth.

Pesticides

The pesticides referred to here are located under your sink or in the garden shed. Insect repellents for both home and garden are as deadly to your health as they are for the creature you are killing off. Lawn-care chemicals were targeted by the National Cancer Institute in a 1987 study showing that children from households who routinely sprayed their lawns were nine times more likely to develop leukemia.

One good reason not to have insect repellents in your home is to prevent your children from drinking them. There are 2.5 million poisonings a year in America from ingesting these household pesticides. You can easily go green by using natural products to prevent infestation:

◆ Ants: Finally there's a good use for aspartame, an artificial sweetener that goes under the names Nutrasweet and Equal. It's a great ant killer! Pick some up at the grocery store and sprinkle some near the area you find the ants. They will take it back to their nest, effectively killing them off. Keep out of reach of children and adults.

◆ Earwigs and grain bugs: Place bay leaves in the jars you store your grains and bugs will stay out. You can also place the dried leaves around your home to help keep bugs away.

◆ Mice: Here's a good one—mice cannot tolerate the smell of mint. Make some mint tea and soak cotton balls or cloth and leave near their entry point.

◆ Bees and wasps: In a spray bottle combine equal parts laundry detergent and water. In the evening, while the wasps are resting, spray the nest. Avoid spraying during the day when they can defend themselves.

Boric acid, or Borax, is the safest of all the natural pesticides. You can use it against invasive insects such as cockroaches, ants, fleas, water bugs, silverfish, palmetto bugs, and termites. Mixed with diluted hydrogen peroxide, it works against all forms of fungus and mold, including the dreaded "black mold." It is mined from the Mojave desert, then ground into a fine white powder. It is not a hazardous chemical and is safe to have around your children and pets.

Air Purifiers

There are any number of air purifiers on the market, so choosing one can be confusing. Plus, they often wear a big price tag. Keep in mind that this machine will effectively purify the air in your home by keeping toxic fumes and particles out of the air. Look for one that will cover the square footage of your home and does not need a lot of filter changes. Some brand name purifiers have radiant catalytic ionization, used by NASA to scrub the air inside a spacecraft.

Basically, you want an air purifier that will eliminate odors, kill airborne germs, and improve the quality of your indoor air without making too much noise. Test it first before buying.

Alternative Building Materials

This topic is a whole world in itself. We are surrounded by toxic chemical fumes from carpets and furniture, and we build our homes and offices with toxic materials.

Detox Alert _____

One of the most dangerous heavy metals is mercury, which is used in thermostats; switches; gas and water flow meters; boilers; standing pilot lights; and fluorescent, compact fluorescent, and high-intensity discharge lamps.

According to green building specialist Cameron Lory, 92 percent of persistent, bioaccumulative, and toxic (PBT) chemicals leave manufacturing facilities through products shipped to consumers, not through emissions out of smokestacks. These include building products, such as HVAC components, lighting systems, textiles and furnishings, roofing, pipes, and interior finishes.

Bromated flame retardants are emitted from drapes, upholstery, furniture, and electronic products. Then there is polyvinyl chloride (PVC), which releases dioxin, hexachlorobenzene, metal stabilizers, and phathalates in flooring, carpet backing, shower curtains, acoustical ceiling tiles, window and door frames, water pipes, and home siding.

Alternative building materials such as water-based adhesives, low-VOC paints, and nontoxic insulation foam are available and are being used more often as consumers demand them. It is best to educate yourself on the topic and go totally alternative in your choices. Otherwise, one wrong decision, whether in choosing a toxic glue or paint, can eliminate the health benefits of the other materials you choose.

Low VOC Paints

VOC stands for volatile organic compounds, found in the oil-based and latex paints we spread across our walls and buildings. It is toxic to your health, especially as the VOC rating gets higher, and contributes to global warming. New EPA "smog" regulations are affecting the use of high VOC content paint. As the VOCs volatilize, the gas reacts with sunlight and fossil fuel combustion by-products to form ozone and smog. The California Air Resources Board estimates 100 million pounds of VOCs are released into the air annually.

When painting inside or outside your home, choose water-based paints with a low or no VOC emission. Many paint companies now make these paints, so you won't have a problem getting the color you love without having to suffer the toxic paint fumes.

Your Energy Use

Here's where the footprint you leave on the earth has a major impact. As third-world populations advance their lifestyles, more carbon emissions will enter the atmosphere. Their use of electricity combined with your use is the largest producer of those carbon emissions. Small things that you do can make a major difference, and if you encourage others to do the same, it can have a huge impact on the way our climate is going.

Take, for instance, the light bulbs you use in your home. According to the Department of Energy, if every household in America changed just one light bulb to a compact fluorescent bulb, enough energy would be saved to light 7 million homes. This would also reduce greenhouse gas emissions equivalent to 1 million cars. That's by changing just one light bulb!

Here are 12 suggestions from www.carbonfootprint.com that you can use, beginning today:

1. Change over to renewable sources of electricity such as wind or solar power.
2. Turn off lights and appliances when not being used.
3. Turn down the central heating 3°F to 4°F.
4. Turn down the water heating setting just 2 degrees.
5. Check the central heating timer setting so as not to overheat your house when no one is home.
6. Fill your dishwasher and washing machine with a full load to save water, electricity, and detergent.
7. Fill the kettle with only as much water as you need.
8. Unplug your mobile phone as soon as it has finished charging.
9. Defrost your fridge/freezer regularly.
10. Do your weekly shopping in a single trip.
11. Hang out the washing to dry rather than tumble drying it.
12. Go for a walk/run rather than drive to the gym.

 Healthy Tidbits

Keep your car in top running order with regular tune-ups and full tires so it will consume less gas.

Drive Less

Regardless of the cost of gas, the emissions continue to pollute the air and burn up precious natural resources. Rather than drive to work, carpool with others, take a bus or train, work from home, and plan to buy a hybrid car. If you haven't been on a bicycle in years, there's no better time than the present. You can find a good used bicycle at garage sales or through newspaper ads. Outfit it with a basket and use it as your local transportation.

America loves automobiles, and they are hard to give up for something as slow as a bicycle. But if you live in an area that you can safely go from town to home using peddle energy, it will provide you with daily exercise and contribute to helping the planet.

Home Insulation

Making a few changes in how you insulate your home can help cut down on electricity expenditures. You can do this by:

- Insulating the walls in your home.
- Insulating the hot-water tank.
- Insulating the roof with loft insulation.
- Installing energy-efficient windows.
- Using shades or curtains to block sun and cold.
- Closing off unused rooms.
- Installing a programmable thermostat.
- Installing fans instead of air-conditioning.

Maybe you can't do it all at once, but little by little if you can get one thing changed at a time, your initial investment will have paid for itself after a few years of lower energy bills.

Sick Building Syndrome

Now, let's take all the chemicals you have just been reading about in this chapter, put them in an office space without adequate ventilation, and sit you in the middle of it all, day after day. The building may be sick, but eventually it is your health that will be affected.

It is the elevated levels of carbon dioxide, chemicals, cleaning solutions, office machinery, and any fungus or mold growing in the walls that gives it the name "sick building syndrome." What happens to you is another story. Symptoms for multiple chemical sensitivity include a rapid heart rate, chest pain, sweating, shortness of breath, fatigue, flushing, dizziness, nausea, choking, trembling, numbness, coughing, hoarseness, and difficulty concentrating. You can say it's because you don't like your job, but unless you remove yourself from that environment, your symptoms will only get worse.

> **Pure Insights**
>
> My condition [burning eyes and lungs, headaches, skin rash, and loss of concentration] was caused by invisible volatile gases that leach from new synthetic carpets, wall coverings, and most office furniture. Also known as "multiple chemical sensitivity," sick building syndrome is characterized by the loss of the body's ability to handle synthetic chemicals.
>
> —Greg Horn, *Living Green*

The Least You Need to Know

- Every purchase you make has an impact on the economy, health, and environment of your country and ultimately the world.

- Make eating organically each day a top priority.

- All-purpose cleaners can cause irritation to your eyes and skin, and inhaling the fumes can harm your lungs. Look for natural alternatives instead.

- If you consider all the fabrics, skin-care lotions, and detergents you use each day, you might be surprised at the level of chemicals you could be absorbing.

- Committing to a few small changes each month can make a big impact on the health of the environment.

- With sick building syndrome, your body has lost the ability to tolerate synthetic chemicals.

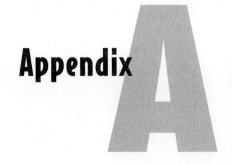

Appendix A

Daily Checklists

Weeks One and Five

This is a helpful way to keep track of all the foods and supplements you need to be taking on a daily basis. You can make a copy of this list for each day of the week and keep it handy for making notes.

(Check a box for each serving or activity.)

Have you had:

Morning lemon water: ❑

5 servings of veggies: ❑ ❑ ❑ ❑ ❑

2 servings of fruits: ❑ ❑

1 vegetarian meal: ❑

Omega-3 fatty acids (flax and/or fish oil): ❑ ❑

1–2 enzymes with each meal: ❑ ❑ ❑ ❑

1 green drink: ❑

Probiotics A.M. and P.M.: ❑ ❑

Walking or aerobic-style exercise: ❑

10 minutes of quiet meditation: ❑

30–60 minutes of yoga: ❑

Notes:

_____

_____

_____

_____

Weeks Two and Four

(Check a box for each serving or activity.)

Have you had:

Morning lemon water: ❑

5 servings of veggies: ❑ ❑ ❑ ❑ ❑

2 servings of fruits: ❑ ❑

1 vegetarian meal: ❑

Omega-3 fatty acids (flax and/or fish oil): ❑ ❑

Fiber drink in A.M.: ❑

1–2 enzymes with each meal: ❑ ❑ ❑ ❑

4 servings of green vegetables: ❑ ❑ ❑ ❑

1 serving of fresh vegetable juice: ❑

1 green drink: ❑

Probiotics A.M. and P.M.: ❑ ❑

Walking or aerobic-style exercise: ❑

10 minutes of quiet meditation: ❑

30–60 minutes of yoga or stretching: ❑

Notes:

_____

_____

_____

_____

Recipes

Chapter 9

Tofu Nut Butter

Makes 1 cup

6 TB. roasted almond butter

2 TB. raw, unrefined honey

2 TB. fresh lemon juice

2 TB. white miso

½ lb. firm tofu

Combine the almond butter, honey, lemon juice, miso, and tofu in a food processor and purée until smooth. Serve on spelt crackers or with carrots and celery.

Grilled Chicken with Pesto

Serves 2

⅓ cup walnuts

2 cloves fresh garlic

1 bunch basil leaves

1 cup parsley, tops only

1 tsp. sea salt

⅔ cup extra-virgin olive oil

2 boneless, skinless chicken breasts

In a food processor, chop the walnuts until finely ground, add the garlic and pulse several times. Add the basil, parsley, salt, and half the oil. Purée and slowly add the remaining oil in a stream while machine is running. Add more oil depending on the desired consistency.

Cook the chicken on a grill or in a sauté pan. Serve topped with the pesto.

Watercress Mesclun Salad with Maple Balsamic Vinaigrette

Serves 2

2 bunches watercress

Handful mesclun salad mix

1 carrot, grated

½ cup toasted walnuts

Wash and stem the watercress and place in a salad bowl with the mesclun. Arrange the salad plates and start with the watercress, then mesclun, the grated carrot, and walnuts. Drizzle with warm Maple Balsamic Vinaigrette and serve. Top with protein of choice.

Maple Balsamic Vinaigrette

Makes 1 cup

¼ cup balsamic vinegar

⅔ cup extra-virgin olive oil

1 tsp. maple syrup

Combine the balsamic vinegar, extra-virgin olive oil, and maple syrup in a saucepan and heat until just warm. Serve over salad.

Rosemary Balsamic Chicken Kabobs

Serves 2

¼ cup balsamic vinegar

2 TB. extra-virgin olive oil

2 tsp. organic garlic powder

½ tsp. sea salt

2 boneless, skinless chicken breasts, cubed

1 zucchini, cut into rounds

1 onion, cut into large pieces

Baby bella mushrooms, cleaned

8 wooden skewers, soaked in water before using

Combine the balsamic vinegar, extra-virgin olive oil, garlic powder, and salt in a bowl. Toss the chicken and vegetables in the marinade, cover, and refrigerate for an hour. Thread the chicken and vegetables on the skewers. Cook on a grill or broil in the oven until tender and chicken is cooked through.

Watercress Pomegranate Salad

Serves 2

2 bunches watercress

1 pomegranate

1 carrot, grated

$\frac{1}{3}$ cup toasted pecans

Wash and stem the watercress and place in a salad bowl. Peel and break the pomegranate into individual seeds in a separate bowl. Arrange the salad plates and start with the watercress, then add the grated carrot and pomegranate seeds, and sprinkle with pecans. Top with warm Maple Balsamic Vinaigrette (see earlier recipe) and serve.

Kale Walnut Salad

Serves 2

1 bunch organic kale, trimmed

$\frac{1}{2}$ cup fennel bulb, chopped

$\frac{1}{3}$ cup walnuts, toasted

2 stalks green onion, chopped

In a large skillet or saucepan, place $\frac{1}{4}$-inch water and add the kale. Cover and bring to a boil. Reduce heat and simmer until tender, about five minutes. When tender, cool, chop, and place in a salad bowl. Add the fennel, walnuts, and green onion. Toss with a lemon oil vinaigrette. Serve with grilled lamb chops.

Chapter 10

Tahini Lemon Dressing

Makes ½ cup

2 TB. tahini
Juice of ½ lemon
1 tsp. white miso
⅓ cup water

Purée the tahini, lemon, white miso, and water in a blender until smooth.

Soft Brown Rice and Quinoa

Makes 5 cups

½ cup brown rice
½ cup quinoa
5 cups water
½ tsp. sea salt

The night before serving, combine the brown rice, quinoa, water, and sea salt in a 3-quart slow cooker and cook overnight on low. Serve warm with toasted pumpkin seeds and cooked kale.

Eggs Florentine

Serves 1

1 mochi waffle

1 cup cooked spinach

1 egg, poached or soft-boiled

Salt and pepper

Toast and lightly butter the mochi waffle, then top with spinach and egg. Season to taste with salt and pepper.

Chicken Garlic Soup

Makes about 10 cups

5 whole garlic cloves

1 cup baby carrots

1 sweet potato, peeled and cubed

1 TB. ginger, minced

2 cups chicken, cubed

1 tsp. dried basil

8 cups vegetable stock or water

Sea salt to taste

Place all ingredients in a slow cooker and cook on low for four to six hours, or until chicken is done and vegetables are tender. Freeze leftovers for a future meal. (Vegetarians can replace the chicken with chickpeas.)

Risotto with Wild Mushrooms

Serves 4

½ cup dried wild mushrooms

½ onion, chopped

2 TB. extra-virgin olive oil

2 cloves garlic, minced

1 cup uncooked brown rice

2 cups vegetable broth (include soaking broth)

1 tsp. sea salt

1 cup cannellini beans

Soak the mushrooms in a bowl with 1 cup of water for 15 minutes. When done, drain and reserve the soaking liquid. In a Dutch oven, sauté the onion in oil and add the garlic, soaked mushrooms, and rice. Add the vegetable broth plus mushroom-soaking liquid, and sea salt. Reduce heat and simmer until water is absorbed. When done, fold in the beans. Spoon into a bowl and top with steamed spinach and toasted pine nuts.

Roasted Salmon

Serves 2

Extra-virgin olive oil

2 salmon fillets

Sea salt

1 bunch escarole, cooked

Preheat oven to 450°F. Heat cast-iron skillet over medium/high heat. When hot, brush with a generous coating of olive oil. Lightly sprinkle the salmon with sea salt. Sear the fillets skin side up for two minutes. When golden brown, transfer to oven for three to six minutes until fish becomes translucent. Transfer salmon to serving dish with cooked escarole topped with Lemon Garlic Sauce (see next page).

Lemon Garlic Sauce

Makes ¼ cup

1 clove garlic
½ cup fresh parsley
2 TB. fresh lemon juice
2 TB. extra-virgin olive oil

In food processor, add garlic and parsley and process. Drizzle lemon juice and olive oil through the feed tube while food processor is running.

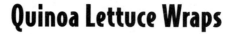

Quinoa Lettuce Wraps

Serves 2

½ cup cooked quinoa
2 TB. chopped fresh parsley
1 clove garlic, minced
Juice of ½ lemon
1 tsp. extra-virgin olive oil
½ cup cooked chickpeas
1 grated carrot
4 large red lettuce leaves

Combine all ingredients except red lettuce. Mix well. Lay out lettuce leaf and spoon quinoa mixture toward end of leaf. Roll up and place on plate. Roll the remaining leaves.

Vegetable Shish Kabobs

Serves 4

3 cloves garlic, minced
Pinch of stevia
4 TB. coconut milk
1 TB. medium curry paste
½ tsp. sea salt
1 tsp. ground cumin
1 tsp. ground turmeric
1 tsp. grated ginger
1 container organic extra-firm tofu, sliced
2 zucchini, cut into 1-inch rounds
1 large onion, cut into chunks
1 red pepper, cut into chunks
12 wooden skewers, soaked in water before using

Combine garlic, stevia, coconut milk, curry paste, and spices in a jar and shake well. In a covered container, place the sliced tofu and cover with marinade. Refrigerate for several hours or overnight. Thread the vegetables onto wooden skewers, alternating the vegetables and tofu. Brush with the marinade and grill until veggies are soft and the tofu is browned.

Chapter 12

Arame and Brown Rice

Serves 4

$\frac{1}{2}$ **cup arame**

2 cups cooked brown rice

2 green onions, sliced

1 carrot, shredded

1 tsp. olive oil or flaxseed oil

Sea salt and cayenne pepper

Soak the arame for 10 minutes. Drain and bring a small pot of water to a boil. Add the arame and simmer another 10 minutes. Drain and fold into cooked rice. Add the green onions, carrot, and oil. Season to taste with salt and cayenne pepper.

To complete this dish, top it with sautéed kale, cooked navy beans, and toasted pumpkin seeds.

Glossary

acidophilus   Milk fermented using bacterial cultures; used to treat digestive disorders.

allergy   A hypersensitivity to a specific substance (food, pollen, dust, etc.) or condition (heat or cold).

allopathic   The treatment of disease using conventional medical therapies, as opposed to the use of alternative medical or nonconventional therapies.

antibiotics   Any of certain substances, such as penicillin or streptomycin, produced by various microorganisms and capable of destroying or weakening bacteria.

antigen   A substance to which the body reacts by producing antibodies.

antioxidants   Substances that retard the body's normal process of oxidation, meaning a reaction to oxygen that releases free radicals that damage cells and break the body down.

aromatherapy   The use of essential oils and other scented compounds made from plant material for the purpose of affecting a person's mood or improving his or her health.

ayurvedic medicine   An ancient system of health care that is native to the Indian subcontinent.

bifidophilus   Beneficial microflora for the intestines.

bioflavonoids   The natural pigments of fruits and vegetables that have numerous benefits.

Candida albicans   An overgrowth of yeast organisms in the large intestine. They feed on sugar, refined carbohydrates, fermented foods, alcohol, and dairy products.

carcinogen   Any substance that causes cancer.

carotenoids   The pigments that protect dark-green, yellow, orange, and red fruits and vegetables from sun damage and work as antioxidants in humans.

cellulite   The protrusion of subcutaneous fat into the dermis, creating a rippling, lumpy appearance to the skin.

chelation therapy   A process involving the use of chelating agents to remove heavy metals from the body.

diuretic   Any substance that increases the flow of urine.

flavonoids   A class of plant secondary metabolites most commonly known for their antioxidant activity. Also commonly referred to as bioflavonoids.

free radicals   Toxins produced as a result of accumulated harm from ongoing chemical reactions within cells, which ultimately damage cells and cause a person to age.

glycation   The uncontrolled reaction of sugars with proteins. Causing damage to be done to critical proteins of long-lived nerve cells in aging.

hepatic   Medical term used in reference to the liver.

hepatic artery   The artery that brings blood into the liver.

holistic medicine   Medical care that views physical, mental, and spiritual aspects of life as closely interconnected and balanced.

lumen of the intestines   The space inside any tubular structure in the body (for example, an intestine, artery, or vein).

miso   Fermented soybean paste high in enzymes.

MSG (monosodium glutamate)   Manufactured/processed free glutamic acid. It is present in most processed foods.

mochi   A Japanese product made by pounding sweet rice.

nephritis   Inflammation of the kidneys.

onychomycosis   A fungus that feeds on the keratin, which makes up the surface of your toenail.

ozonator   A device with an aerator at the end of its hose that is inserted into food, oil, or water. The purpose is to sanitize and oxidize by adding a tiny amount of ozone. Ozonation quickly kills bacteria and viruses in food and beverages.

Patanjali's sutras   A collection of guidelines in the form of a manual, which detail the path to liberation based on The Eight-Limb Path of yoga.

peristaltic action   The way the intestines move waste through the colon.

pharmacopeia   Official books of drugs and medicines.

phytonutrients   Plant-derived compounds that are believed to improve your health, but aren't essential to your health.

polyphenols   A group of chemical substances found in plants, characterized by the presence of more than one phenol group per molecule.

portal vein   The vein that transports blood from the gastrointestinal track to the liver.

prana   A Sanskrit word that translates as both "breath" and "life." Prana is the vital energy force that pervades our physical, mental, and spiritual bodies, keeping us alive and vibrant.

pressing   A form of cooking raw vegetables using salt and pressure. It helps you more easily digest the vegetables and gives them a wonderful texture and quality.

probiotics   Dietary supplements containing potentially beneficial microflora bacteria.

REM sleep   A stage of sleep that recurs several times during the night and is marked by dreaming, rapid-eye movements (REM) under closed lids, and elevated pulse rate and brain activity.

renal calculi   Hard masses of mineral salts that form in the urinary tract and restrict urine flow.

risk assessment   The evaluation of the quantity of a toxic substance deemed safe in the environment and water supply.

sluggish colon   A buildup of putrid waste products leading to constipation.

spastic colon   A condition of the bowel in which there is recurrent pain with constipation or diarrhea, or alternating attacks of these.

Spirulina algae   A microscopic blue-green algae that exists as a single-celled organism, turning sunlight into life energy.

synergy   The phenomenon in which the combined action of two things—for example, drugs and muscles—is greater than their effects individually.

tincture   A medicinal substance in an alcoholic solution.

vitamins   Nutrients considered essential to health; a shortage of vitamins can create health problems.

Appendix D

Resources

This resource list is provided to help you learn more about how you can maintain a healthy lifestyle and support your local and world community at the same time. There are books to read, websites that educate, and companies you can order healthy products from online. All of this information will contribute to you and your family's better health and well-being.

Books

Aihara, Herman. *Acid & Alkaline*. Oroville, California: George Oshawa Macrobiotic Foundation, 1986.

Baroody, Dr. Theodore A. *Alkalize or Die*. Waynesville, North Carolina: Holographic Health Press, 2002.

Cabot, Dr. Sandra. *The Healthy Liver & Bowel Book*. Scottsdale, Arizona: SCB International Inc., 1999.

Clark, Dr. Hulda. *The Cure for All Cancers*. San Diego, California: ProMotion Publishing, 1993.

D'Adamo, Dr. Peter J., with Catherine Whitney. *Eat Right 4 Your Type: The Individualized Diet Solution to Staying Healthy, Living Longer & Achieving Your Ideal Weight*. New York: G. P. Putnam's Sons, 1996.

Dean, Dr. Carolyn, and Trueman Tuck. *Death by Modern Medicine*. Belleville, Ontario: Matrix Verité, Inc., 2005.

Dries, Jan. *The New Book of Food Combining: A Completely New Approach to Healthy Eating*. Rockport, Massachusetts: Element Books, 1992.

Gates, Donna, and Linda Schatz. *The Body Ecology Diet: Recovering Your Health & Rebuilding Your Immunity*. Atlanta, Georgia: B.E.D. Publications, 1996.

Hills, Hilda Cherry. *Good Food, Milk Free, Grain Free*. New Canaan, Connecticut: Keats Publishing, Inc., 1980.

Horn, Greg. *Living Green: A Practical Guide To Simple Sustainability*. Topanga, California: Freedom Press, 2006.

Kushi, Michio. *How to See Your Health: Book of Oriental Diagnosis*. Tokyo and New York: Japan Publications, 1980.

————. *Macrobiotic Home Remedies*. Tokyo and New York: Japan Publications, 1985.

Pitchford, Paul. *Healing with Whole Foods: Asian Traditions and Modern Nutrition, Third Edition*. Berkeley, California: North Atlantic Books, 2002.

Quigley, Delia. *The Body Rejuvenation Cleanse*. Blairstown, New Jersey: Stillpoint Schoolhouse Publications, 2007.

Rodale Health Books. *The Purification Plan: Clear Your Body of the Toxins That Contribute to Weight Gain, Fatigue, and Chronic Illness*. Emmaus, Pennsylvania: Rodale, Inc., 2005.

Rosenvold, Lloyd. *Can A Gluten-Free Diet Help? How?* New Canaan, Connecticut: Keats Publishing, Inc., 1992.

Wade, Carlson. *Inner Cleansing: How to Free Yourself From Joint-Muscle-Artery-Circulation Sludge*. Paramus, New Jersey: Prentice Hall, 1992.

Wing, R. L. *I Ching, Book of Changes*. New York: Doubleday Main Street Books, 1982.

Reference Articles

"Acute Effects of Dietary Caffeine and Sucrose on Urinary Mineral Excretion in Healthy Adolescents," by L. K. Massey; *Nutritional Research* 8(9), 1988.

"The Effects of Chlorine in Your Water: Chlorine, Cancer and Heart Disease," courtesy of Aquasana; www.healthynewage.com/chlorine-cancer.htm.

"Harmful Teflon Chemical to Be Eliminated by 2015," by Juliet Eilperin; *Washington Post*, January 26, 2006.

"Parasites," by Marcelle Pick; www.womentowomen.com.

"Role of Sugars in Human Neutrophilic Phacocytosis," by A. Sanchez, et al.; *American Journal of Clinical Nutrition* 26:180, 1973.

"Single Strains vs. Probiotic Stews," by Linda Mulder; www.ffnmag.com.

Websites

Supplements and Supplies

Atlantic Spice Company: www.atlanticspice.com

Essential 3 Oils: www.essentialthree.com

Frontier Essential Oils: www.frontiercoop.com

Herbalist and Alchemist: www.herbalist-alchemist.com

Mountain Rose Herbs: www.mountainroseherbs.com

Nature's Sunshine: www.naturessunshine.com

Simplers Botanical Company: www.simplers.com/herbal/organic.htm

Young Living Essential Oils: www.youngliving.us

To Order Organic Detox Foods

All-organic food, Diamond Organics: www.diamondorganics.com

Alternative and herbal therapeutic products, Dr. Joseph Mercola: www.mercola.com

Coffee (organic, sustainably grown, fair trade), Green Mountain Coffee Roasters: www.greenmountaincoffee.com

Frozen fruits and vegetables, Cascadian Farms: www.cfarm.com

Holistic health products, The Kushi Institute: www.kushistore.com/acatalog/welcome.html

Nature's Harvest, PO Box 291, 28 Main St., Blairstown, NJ 07825. Contact Michelle St. Andre: 908-362-6766; Harvest6766@embarqmail.com

Organic tomato sauces and salsas, Seeds of Change: www.seedsofchange.com

Vegetables, Earthbound Farm: www.ebfarm.com

Energy Consumption Statistics

Energy Information Administration website: www.eia.doe.gov/kids/classactivities/CrunchTheNumbersIntermediateDec2002.pdf

Saving with Compact Fluorescents, Environmental Defense: www.environmentaldefense.org/article.cfm?contentid=5215

Saving with Recycling, National Resources Defense Council: www.nrdc.org/land/forests/gtissue.asp

U.S. Department of Energy website: www.energy.gov

U.S. Department of Energy's Division of Energy Efficiency and Renewable Energy: www.eere.energy.gov

Sustainable Building and Retrofitting

Alternative energy systems, products, and installation: www.utilityfree.com

Bob Swain: www.bobswain.com

General building information: www.greenbuilder.com

Saline Pool Systems: www.salinepoolsystems.com

Sick Building Syndrome: www.wellbuilding.com

Renewable Resource Programs and Information

Green-e program, the nation's leading independent certification and verification program: www.green-e.org

Green Facts provides factual information on health and the environment: www.greenfacts.org

Spirituality

Essene Gospels of Peace: www.essene.com/GospelOfPeace/peace1.html

Genesis Farm, a learning center for Earth studies: www.genesisfarm.org

Native American spirituality: www.greenspirit.org.uk/Resources/NatAmerSpirit.htm

Other Resources

Calculate your carbon footprint: www.carbonfootprint.com or www.greentagusa.org

Cleaning Chemicals: www.restoreproducts.com

Daliya Robson's website for nontoxic household furnishings: www.nontoxic.com

Dangers of Teflon: www.tuberose.com/Teflon.html

Environmental building supplies: www.greendepot.com

Food safety information: www.organicconsumers.org

For hydrotherapy: Living Waters Wellness Center, www.colonhealthnj.com

For sustainably harvested household products: www.seventhgeneration.com

Monosodium Glutamate (MSG) website: www.truthinlabeling.org

Index

Q-R

qi, 184
quinoa, 114-115
  benefits of, 83
  cooking times, 116

radishes
  benefits of, 83
  Spinach Arugula Salad, 198
raw honey, 118
raw vegetables, pressing, 196
Raw-Food Fast, 150-153
recipes
  Cooked Brown Rice, 190
  Dandelion Watercress Pressed Salad, 197
  Detox Pesto Sauce, 199
  Dr. Hulda Clark's Gallbladder Flush, 216-217
  facial masks, 239-241
  facials, 239
  ginger compresses, 230
  Lemon Miso Dressing, 197
  Lemonade Recipe, 147
  Maple Lemon Dressing, 151
  natural exfoliants, 245
  Olive Oil Lemon Flush, 220-221
  peppermint soaks, 243
  Potassium Broth, 106
  Sea Salt Scrub, 255
  spa baths, 246
  Spinach Arugula Salad, 198
  Tomato Herb Dressing, 151
refined sugar, 35
  eliminating, 114
refined wheat flour, 34
reflexology, 143, 255-256
religious food customs, 263-264
renal calculi, 225
rest, importance of, 144
retracing, 102
Reuben, David, 41

ribonucleotides, 26
rice, brown rice, benefits of, 189
rice syrup, 118
roasting
  nuts, 117
  seeds, 117
rosemary, benefits of, 246
rye, 114

S

saccharin, 27
SAD (Standard American Diet), 34-35
sage, 91
salad dressings
  Carrot Ginger Dressing, 152
  Lemon Miso Dressing, 197
  Maple Lemon Dressing, 151
  Tomato Herb Dressing, 151
salad greens, benefits of, 83
salads
  Dandelion Watercress Pressed Salad, 197
  Spinach Arugula Salad, 198
salty flavors, 171
Samadhi (self-realization), 265
saturated fats, 117
Saturday (weekend detox program), 200
sauces, Detox Pesto Sauce, 199
saunas, benefits of, 143, 250-252
Schlosser, Eric, 35
Sea Salt Scrubs, 255
sea vegetables, 158-159
  benefits of, 83
seasonal detoxification, 181-182
  Autumn, 187-189
  Five Element theory, 182-184
  Spring, 184
  Summer, 185-187
  Winter, 189-192
Seaweed Body Wraps, 255
second week (detox program), 127
  foods to eliminate, 128-130
  meals and snacks, 135-138

Take care of your body with help

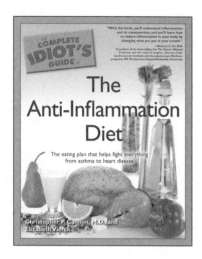

ISBN: 978-1-59257-558-9

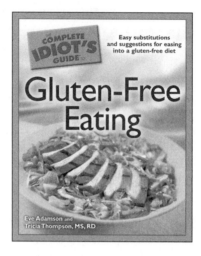

ISBN: 978-1-59257-683-8

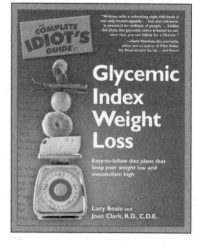

ISBN: 978-1-59257-404-9

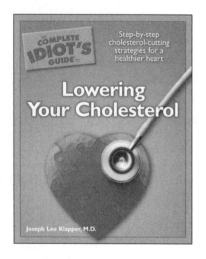

ISBN: 978-1-59257-552-7

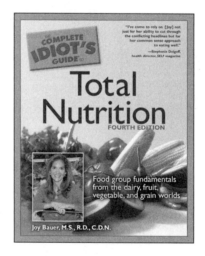

ISBN: 978-1-59257-439-1

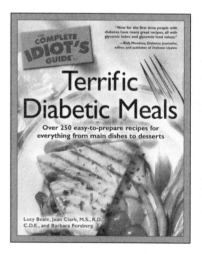

ISBN: 978-1-59257-275-5

from these *Complete Idiot's Guides*®

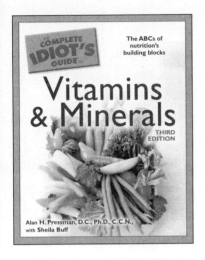

ISBN: 978-1-59257-609-8

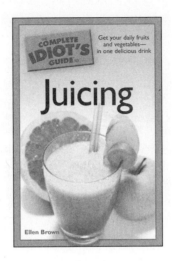

ISBN: 978-1-59257-568-8

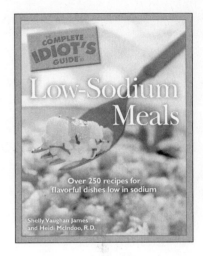

ISBN: 978-1-59257-467-4

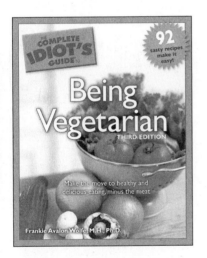

ISBN: 978-1-59257-682-1

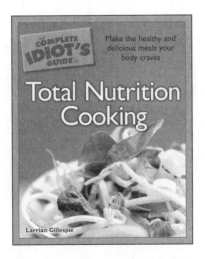

ISBN: 978-1-59257-549-7

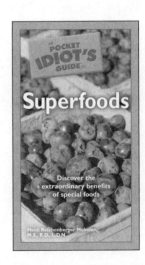

ISBN: 978-1-59257-612-8

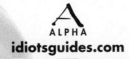

CHECK OUT THESE BEST-SELLERS

More than 450 titles available at booksellers and online retailers everywhere!

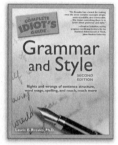

978-1-59257-115-4

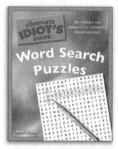

978-1-59257-900-6

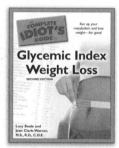

978-1-59257-855-9

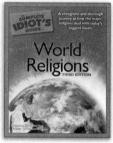

978-1-59257-222-9

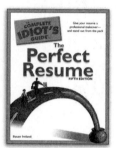

978-1-59257-957-0

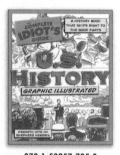

978-1-59257-785-9

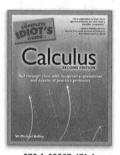

978-1-59257-471-1

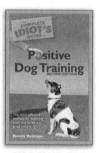

978-1-59257-483-4

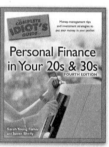

978-1-59257-883-2

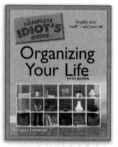

978-1-59257-966-2

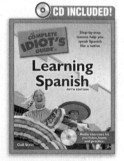

978-1-59257-908-2

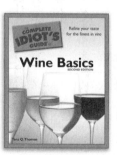

978-1-59257-786-6

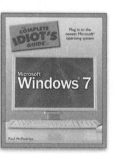

978-1-59257-954-9

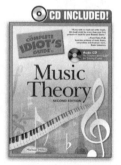

978-1-59257-437-7

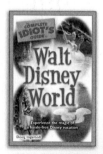

978-1-59257-888-7

ALPHA   idiotsguides.com